PUBLIC HEALTH IN THE 21ST CENTURY

PHARMACOTHERAPY OF SMOKING CESSATION: CURRENT AND FUTURE STATUS

Public Health in the 21st Century

Additional books in this series can be found on Nova's website under the Series tab.

Additional E-books in this series can be found on Nova's website under the E-book tab.

Substance Abuse Assessment, Interventions and Treatment

Additional books in this series can be found on Nova's website under the Series tab.

Additional E-books in this series can be found on Nova's website under the E-book tab.

Public Health in the 21st Century

Pharmacotherapy of Smoking Cessation: Current and Future Status

Kiran Sondhi

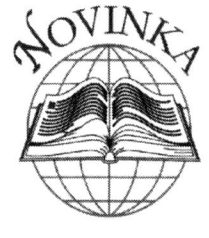

Nova Science Publishers, Inc.
New York

Copyright © 2010 by Nova Science Publishers, Inc.

All rights reserved. No part of this book may be reproduced, stored in a retrieval system or transmitted in any form or by any means: electronic, electrostatic, magnetic, tape, mechanical photocopying, recording or otherwise without the written permission of the Publisher.

For permission to use material from this book please contact us:
Telephone 631-231-7269; Fax 631-231-8175
Web Site: http://www.novapublishers.com

NOTICE TO THE READER

The Publisher has taken reasonable care in the preparation of this book, but makes no expressed or implied warranty of any kind and assumes no responsibility for any errors or omissions. No liability is assumed for incidental or consequential damages in connection with or arising out of information contained in this book. The Publisher shall not be liable for any special, consequential, or exemplary damages resulting, in whole or in part, from the readers' use of, or reliance upon, this material. Any parts of this book based on government reports are so indicated and copyright is claimed for those parts to the extent applicable to compilations of such works.

Independent verification should be sought for any data, advice or recommendations contained in this book. In addition, no responsibility is assumed by the publisher for any injury and/or damage to persons or property arising from any methods, products, instructions, ideas or otherwise contained in this publication.

This publication is designed to provide accurate and authoritative information with regard to the subject matter covered herein. It is sold with the clear understanding that the Publisher is not engaged in rendering legal or any other professional services. If legal or any other expert assistance is required, the services of a competent person should be sought. FROM A DECLARATION OF PARTICIPANTS JOINTLY ADOPTED BY A COMMITTEE OF THE AMERICAN BAR ASSOCIATION AND A COMMITTEE OF PUBLISHERS.

Additional color graphics may be available in the e-book version of this book.

LIBRARY OF CONGRESS CATALOGING-IN-PUBLICATION DATA

Sondhi, Kiran.
 Pharmacotherapy of smoking cessation : current and future status /
Authors, Kiran Sondhi.
     p. cm.
 Includes index.
 ISBN 978-1-61761-601-3 (softcover)
 1. Nicotine addiction--Treatment. 2. Nicotine--Physiological effect. 3. Smoking cessation. I. Title.
 RC567.S68 2011
 616.86'5061--dc22
                                                                    2010031200

Published by Nova Science Publishers, Inc. † New York

CONTENTS

Preface		vii
Chapter 1	Neurobiology of Nicotine Dependence	1
Chapter 2	Pharmacotherapy	3
Chapter 3	Nicotine Replacement Therapy (NRT)	5
Chapter 4	Nicotine Gum	7
Chapter 5	Transdermal Nicotine Patch	11
Chapter 6	Nicotine Lozenge	13
Chapter 7	Nicotine Nasal Spray	15
Chapter 8	Nicotine Inhaler	19
Chapter 9	Status and Newer Recommendations for NRT	21
Chapter 10	Bupropion	25
Chapter 11	Varenicline	27
Chapter 12	Clonidine	29
Chapter 13	Nortriptyline	31
Chapter 14	Nicotinic or Non-Nicotinic Therapies under Investigation	33
Chapter 15	Rimonabant	35
Chapter 16	Mecamylamine	37
Chapter 17	Inhibitors of Nicotine Metabolism	39

Chapter 18	Opioid Antagonists	41
Chapter 19	Antidepressants	43
Chapter 20	GABAergic Agents	45
Chapter 21	Drug Therapy in Pregnant Females	47
Chapter 22	Critical Issues of Pharmacotherapy	49
References		51
Index		65

PREFACE

Realizing the impact of smoking on the human beings, the US Public Health Service updated its 2000 Guidelines for Treating Tobacco Use and Dependence in 2008[1] and the WHO released the MPOWER package [2] Both the guidelines aim to counter the tobacco epidemic and reduce its deadly toll. Smoking is a leading preventable cause of mortality in US and worldwide.[3,4] Cigarette smoking is one of the few causes of mortality that are increasing. It is a risk factor for six out of eight leading causes of death in the world and hence contributes to high mortality rate.[2] Smoking prevalence and associated premature mortality varies widely across countries. The prevalence is declining in developed countries and increasing in economically developing nations.[2] Each year, an estimated 443,000 people die of smoking related diseases in the United States.[3,4] In Australia, tobacco smoking is responsible for deaths of 16,000 Australians every year.[5] In United States smoking results in more than $193 billion in medical costs and productivity losses annually.[6] Tobacco use is growing fastest in the low income countries due to steady population growth coupled with tobacco industry targeting; ensuing that millions of people get fatally addicted every year. As many as 100 million Chinese men currently under age 30 will die from tobacco use.[7] In India, about a quarter of deaths among middle-aged men are caused by smoking.[8]

Although smoking rates are declining in US, yet, more and more young adults and children are becoming fresh smokers every day. Each day about 4000 youth ages 12 to 17 years smoke their first cigarette and about 1200 children and adolescents daily become cigarettes smokers.[1] The data made available through litigation has shown that tobacco industry has invested much time and money studying young adult smoking patterns.

The health benefits of smoking cessation are well documented. Smokers who quit reduce their risk of cardiovascular disease, lung disease and cancer and substantially increase their life-expectancy.[9] The US Public Health Service Guideline for treating Tobacco Use and Dependence 2008 Update has re-emphasized the importance of interventions required for successful smoking cessation regimens.[1] In the US, approximately 70% of smokers want to stop smoking and 44% attempt to stop smoking every year. Unfortunately, these efforts are usually unaided and unsuccessful; only approximately 4% to 7% of smokers who attempt to stop smoking are able to do so by themselves.[10]

Drug dependence is a chronic, relapsing disorder in which compulsive drug-seeking and drug-taking behavior persists despite serious negative consequences. Nicotine is the principal component of tobacco smoke that leads to addiction.[11] Nicotine leads to reward and reinforcement, as well as the withdrawal manifestations which further causes negative reinforcement.[12] Cigarette smoking produces high concentrations of nicotine in blood that are comparable to those seen after intravenous administration.

Chapter 1

NEUROBIOLOGY OF NICOTINE DEPENDENCE

Nicotine has both central and peripheral effects. The central effects are complex and remain consistent with repeated dosage whereas the peripheral effects decline on repeated use.[13] At the cellular level in the CNS, , nicotine acts on nicotinic acetylcholine receptors (nAChRs). In the mammalian brain there are as many as nine α subunits ($α_2$ to $α_{10}$) and three β subunits ($β_2$ to $β_4$) of the nicotinic receptors. The most abundant receptor subtypes in human brains are $α_4β_2$, $α_3β_4$ and $α_7$ (homomimeric). The $α_4β_2$ receptors are predominantly present in the cortex and hippocampus.

It is postulated that the $α_4β_2$ hetero-oligomeric receptors play pivotal roles in the addictive effects of nicotine. [14-17] Recent work has identified $α_4β_2$ containing channels in the ventral tegmental area (VTA) as the nAChRs that are required for the rewarding effects of nicotine.[18] Stimulation of central nAChRs (mainly $α_4β_2$) by nicotine results in the release of a variety of neurotransmitters in the brain, most importantly dopamine. The activation of the nicotinic receptors increases the activity of the dopaminergic neurons, especially those present in the VTA of the midbrain, leading to an increase in dopamine release in the Nucleus Accumbens (NAcc), which is thought to mediate reward.[13,19] Dopamine release signals a pleasurable experience and is critical to the reinforcing effects.[20]

Other neurotransmitters including nor-epinephrine, acetylcholine, serotonin, GABA, glutamate and endorphins are also released, mediating various behaviors of nicotine.[22] The addiction to tobacco is more complex than a simple dependence upon nicotine. Two complementary theories have been postulated for the mechanism of dependence. The first theory speculates that smokers maintain $α_4β_2$ nAChRs in a desensitized state to avoid withdrawal.[22] The other theory states that conditioned smoking cues (e.g. taste and feel of the smoke) maintain smoking behavior during periods of saturation and desensitization of brain nAChRs. So, it is thought that smokers continue to smoke throughout the day to maintain plasma nicotine levels that prevent the occurrence of withdrawal symptoms and may also continue to derive some rewarding effects from the conditioned reinforcement associated with smoking.[23] On repeated exposure to nicotine, tolerance or neuroadaptation develops to some effects of nicotine. Concurrently, there is an increase in the number of nAChR binding sites in the brain. This increase represents upregulation in response to desensitization of receptors.

Chapter 2

PHARMACOTHERAPY

The US guidelines[1] and the WHO MPOWER[2] have re-emphasized the role of society, physicians and the drugs in controlling the tobacco epidemic. The guidelines also state that the pharmacotherapy should be offered to "all smokers trying to quit, except in the presence of special circumstances". At present Nicotine Replacement Therapy (NRT) {which includes nicotine gum, nicotine patch, nicotine lozenge, nicotine inhaler and nicotine nasal spray}; Bupropion and Varenicline are approved by FDA for smoking cessation. Other drugs like Clonidine, Nortryptilline are considered appropriate as second line medications for smoking cessation by the Clinical Practice Guidelines on Treating Tobacco Use and Dependence published by the Public Health Service.[1] All the first line and second line agents will be discussed in the following sections. From nearly two decades of experience, it is clear that the currently available medications do not address the needs of all the tobacco users.[24] So, new and old molecules are being investigated for their role in smoking cessation. Many molecules have failed in the early phases of trials whereas few are near approval stage. Most of them have been covered in the following sections. The important ones in this group of drugs include nicotine vaccines, Opioid antagonists- (Naloxone, Naltrexone, Nalmefene); Nicotinic antagonist- (Mecamylamine); Cannabinoid antagonist- (Rimonabant); Antidepressants- (Venlafaxine, Fluoxetine); GABAergic agonists- (Tiagabine and Baclofen); Inhibitors of Nicotine metabolism- (Methoxsalen).

Chapter 3

NICOTINE REPLACEMENT THERAPY (NRT)

Nicotine Replacement Therapy is the most widely studied and used pharmacotherapy for managing nicotine dependence and withdrawal during smoking cessation. The nicotine delivery system itself is an important determinant of the toxic and addictive effects of nicotine use. Therefore, altering the form of nicotine dosing may allow for selective therapeutic action in efforts to develop safer and less addictive nicotine replacement therapies. Nicotine medications act on nAChRs to mimic or replace the effects of nicotine from tobacco smoking. In contrast to smoking, which involves rapid absorption of nicotine, the use of nicotine medications generally provides slower, lower, and less variable plasma nicotine concentrations.[25] Nicotine replacement therapy facilitates smoking cessation by possibly three mechanisms.[22,26] *First and the foremost*, NRT provides an alternative form of nicotine to relieve symptoms of withdrawal in a smoker who is abstaining from tobacco use. Amelioration of these symptoms is observed with relatively low blood levels of nicotine and serves as a counter to negative reinforcement to smoke due to troublesome symptoms. *Second* mechanism is positive reinforcement, particularly for the arousal and stress-relieving effects. The degree of the positive reinforcement is related to the rapidity of absorption and the peak nicotine levels achieved in arterial blood. Positive reinforcement is most relevant to rapid- drug delivery formulations such as nasal spray and to a lesser extent to nicotine gum, inhaler and lozenge. The nicotine patches deliver nicotine gradually, so they do not provide much positive reinforcement. The *third* mechanism is desensitization of the nicotine receptors by nicotine replacement. This leads to a reduced effect of nicotine from cigarettes e.g. when a person smokes a cigarette while on NRT, the puff is less satisfying as it takes out the pleasure of nicotine use and the person is less likely to resume smoking. The onset of action for NRT is not as rapid as that of nicotine obtained through smoking, so the patients become less accustomed to the nearly immediate, reinforcing effects of inhaled tobacco. Most of the studies comparing NRT with placebo have demonstrated a significant improvement over placebo at long term follow-up.[27]

Currently, five formulations of NRT are available either as prescription or OTC drugs in most of the countries. All the NRT products are endorsed by the US Public Health Service Clinical Practice Guideline as first line pharmacotherapies for the treatment of tobacco dependence.[1]

Chapter 4

NICOTINE GUM

Nicotine gum (2 mg) was the first nicotine medication to be approved by FDA in 1984.[25] Today, it is available as an OTC drug in most of the countries. Nicotine gum is a resin complex of nicotine and polacrilin in a chewing gum base that allows for slow release and absorption of nicotine across the oral mucosa. The gum has a distinct, tobacco-like, slightly peppery, minty, or fruity taste and contains buffering agents to increase the salivary pH, which enhances the buccal absorption of nicotine.[28]

About 50% of the nicotine in gum is absorbed through the buccal mucosa.[26] Peak plasma concentrations of nicotine are achieved within approximately 30 minutes of chewing a single piece of gum and then slowly decline thereafter. (Figure 1) The absorption of nicotine gum is reduced with concomitant use of acidic beverages like coffee, tea etc.

The use of nicotine gum increases cessation rates by 50 to 70 percent.[33] Shiffman et al demonstrated that nicotine gum could reduce acute craving following exposure to a provocative stimulus.[34] Some initial reductions in craving are likely due to the behavioral effects of chewing gum. However, after about 15-20 minutes of chewing, the nicotine itself reduces craving.[35]

The gum is available in two doses: 2 mg and 4 mg, delivering approximately 1 mg and 2 mg, respectively. Individuals who smoke <25 cigarettes per day are generally recommended to use the 2 mg strength, and those smoking more should use the 4 mg strength.[1] (Table 1) During the initial 6 weeks of therapy, one piece of gum every 1 to 2 hours should be used while awake. Proper chewing technique (chew and park) is crucial when using the nicotine gum.[28] The chew/park steps should be repeated until most of the nicotine is extracted; this generally occurs after 30 minutes and becomes obvious when chewing no longer elicits the characteristic taste or tingling sensation.

The use of nicotine gum is beneficial for patients who have weight gain concerns, who report boredom as a trigger for smoking, who desire flexibility in dosing and prefer the ability to self-regulate nicotine levels to manage withdrawal symptoms. This is not a formulation of choice for people who find it difficult to use or find chewing the gum socially unacceptable. Nicotine gum should not be used by patients with temporomandibular joint (TMJ) conditions.[28]

ADVERSE EFFECTS

The adverse effects are generally mild and include - mouth soreness, hiccups, dyspepsia and jaw ache. Some of these can be alleviated by adopting proper chewing techniques. The gum placement site within the mouth should be rotated so as to decrease the incidence of oral irritation.

Table 1. Pharmacotherapy for smoking cessation[9]

Drug	Dose	Adverse effects/ drug interactions	Comments
NRT: sustained release Nicotine transdermal patch	>20 cigarettes/day: 1 patch (21 mg/24 h) for 4-6 weeks, then taper to 14 mg/day for 2-4 weeks, then 7 mg/day for 2-4 weeks.	Skin sensitivity and irritation (most common); abnormal dreams; insomnia; nausea, dyspepsia.	Start patch on quit date. Advise not to smoke cigarettes while using the patch, though this is generally safe and does not indicate treatment failure
Nicotine inhaler	At least six doses/day for first 3-6 weeks. Then gradual reduction over next 6-12 weeks; stopping when reduced to 1-2 /day. Maximum 12 g/day	Mild local irritation of mouth and throat, coughing, rhinitis that may decline with continued use.	Not a true inhaler- the nicotine is delivered and absorbed buccally.
Nicotine gum	10-12 pieces/day initially (2mg or 4 mg pieces) to maximum of 20 pieces/day, for 12 weeks. Tapering: 1 piece/day each week, as withdrawal symptoms allow	Moth soreness, hiccups, dyspepsia, jaw ache	4 mg in heavily dependent smokers. Can be used for temporary abstinence.
Nicotine lozenge	1 lozenge (2mg or 4 mg) every 1-2 h upto 6 weeks; every 2-4 h in weeks 7-9; every 4-8 h in weeks 10-12	Nausea, hiccups, heartburn, headache, coughing	
Nicotine nasal spray	1 mg of nicotine nasal spray 1-2 doses/h upto 40 doses/day; for 3 months.	Mild nasal/throat irritation	
Bupropion SR	150 mg daily for 3 days; then 150 mg twice daily for 7-12 weeks. Begin 1-2 weeks before the selected quit date	Insomnia, dry mouth, suicidal tendencies Drug interactions: Clearance may be ↓by inhibitors (e.g. ticlopidine) or↑ by inducers (e.g. phenytoin) of CYP2B6.	Not recommended in patients with conditions predisposing to seizures, history of seizures, current eating disorder or severe hepatic impairment.

Table 1. (Continued).

Drug	Dose	Adverse effects/ drug interactions	Comments
Varenicline	0.5 mg daily for 3 days, then twice daily for 4 days then 1 mg twice daily for 12 weeks. Quit date 1-2 weeks after starting the medication.	Nausea, sleep disturbances, abnormal/vivid /strange dreams.	FDA recommends that patients should inform about any history of psychiatric illness prior to starting medication. Monitoring required.

Chapter 5

TRANSDERMAL NICOTINE PATCH

Nicotine patch is approved as first line medication for treating tobacco use. The nicotine patch is available both as OTC and prescription drug. Transdermal nicotine delivery system consists of an impermeable surface layer, a nicotine reservoir, an adhesive layer and a removable protective liner.

Plasma nicotine levels obtained via transdermal delivery are approximately 50% lower than those achieved with cigarette smoking, but still alleviate the symptoms of withdrawal.[26] Currently, various patch formulations with varied design, strength(21 mg, 14 mg, 7 mg, 15 mg, 10 mg, 5 mg), pharmacokinetics and duration of wear (i.e. 16 and 24 hour wear) are available in the market. The transdermal nicotine patch containing about 25 mg of nicotine per 30 cm^2 thin multilayer film laminate patch, is designed to deliver approximately 15 mg of nicotine to the subject in 16 hours of application (31µg/cm^2/h).[36] Mean plasma concentrations of nicotine increase gradually and reach a broad peak at 8 to 10 hours after transdermal application at any site.[36] (Figure 1) It has been seen that after removal of patch, the plasma concentrations exhibit a transient maintenance, which dissipates within 1 hour and then declines with a mean $t_{1/2}$ of approximately 4 to 5 hours. It has also been demonstrated that the plasma concentrations after application to the upper arm are similar to those of the back but higher compared with the abdomen. The differences in pharmacokinetics have been illustrated in a head-to-head clinical trial.[37] It has been seen that nicotine release from the patch increases during exercise, but this increase has no significant effect on overall plasma pharmacokinetics.[38] A randomized, double-dummy trial comparing the NicoDerm CQ patch (21 mg/24 hours) to the Nicotrol Patch (15 mg/16 hours) has shown that the 21 mg/24 hour patch yielded better control of craving, not only during the morning hours, but also throughout the day and over the 2-week period of abstinence.[39] It has been demonstrated that the pharmacokinetic and hemodynamic effects of a nicotine patch are significantly different between smokers and nonsmokers.[40]

Smokers who use 10 or less cigarettes per day are instructed to begin with the 14 mg patch and those who smoke more than 10 per day are instructed to start with 21 mg.[26] (Table 1) A recent meta-analysis has shown that the start of the patch treatment before the target quit date produces a robust increase in quit rates compared to the current regimens of starting the patch on the target quit date.[41] Higher levels of smoking necessitate the use of higher-strength formulations and a longer duration of therapy.

The advantages of nicotine patch include easy administration, continuous maintenance of reliable moderate blood nicotine levels (about half of those achieved by smoking) and better compliance.[42] Disadvantages of the patch include a high incidence of skin irritation associated with the patch adhesives and the inability to acutely adjust the dose of nicotine to alleviate symptoms of withdrawal and reduce the craving episodes (whereas the other products offer the potential for greater dose control and the ability to prevent relapse by adjusting the dose of nicotine as an when required). To tackle the acute craving episodes and the withdrawal symptoms, the patients can add nicotine gum or nasal spray to their daily therapy of nicotine patch.

ADVERSE EFFECTS

The adverse effects with nicotine patch are local reactions like erythema, burning and pruritius (at the application site), insomnia and vivid dreams. Other less common adverse effects are vivid or abnormal dreams, insomnia and headache. Rotation of the application sites on daily basis minimizes skin irritation.[1,28]

Chapter 6

NICOTINE LOZENGE

Nicotine lozenge is available as an OTC drug in US. The nicotine polacrilex lozenge is a resin complex of nicotine and polacrilin in a sugarfree, light mint, or cherry-flavored lozenge. Like the nicotine gum, the lozenge also contains buffering agents (sodium carbonate and potassium bicarbonate) to increase salivary pH, thereby enhancing buccal absorption of the nicotine.

The nicotine lozenge dissolves completely and delivers approximately 25% more nicotine than does an equivalent dose of nicotine gum.[43] Peak nicotine concentrations of nicotine with the lozenge are achieved after 30 to 60 minutes of use and then slowly decline thereafter.

The product is available in 2- and 4-mg strengths, which are meant to be consumed like hard candy or other medicinal lozenges (i.e. sucked and moved from side to side in the mouth until fully dissolved). (Table 1) Other NRT formulations use the number of cigarettes smoked per day as the basis for dosing whereas the recommended dosage of the nicotine lozenge is based on the time to first cigarette (TTFC) i.e. the need to smoke soon after waking.[28] Based on this method, people who smoke their first cigarette of the day within 30 minutes of waking are considered highly dependent on nicotine as compared to those who smoke their first cigarette more than 30 minutes after waking.

In a double blind, placebo- controlled randomized trial, 2mg and 4 mg preparations of the nicotine lozenge were evaluated for safety and efficacy. Treatment with the nicotine lozenge resulted in significantly greater 28-day abstinence at 6 weeks, for the 2-mg (46.0% vs. 29.7%; odds ratio [OR], 2.10; 95% confidence interval [CI], 1.59-2.79; $P<.001$) and the 4-mg (48.7% vs. 20.8%; OR, 3.69; 95% CI, 2.74-4.96; $P<.001$) lozenges, compared with placebo. Significant treatment effects were maintained for a full year. Smokers who used more lozenges achieved significantly better treatment effects.[44] A recent meta-analysis of five studies using either the nicotine lozenge (nicotine polacrilin) or sublingual tablet (not available in the United States) concluded that the odds of abstinence at 6 or more months was 2.0 with the tablet/lozenge relative to placebo (95% CI, 1.6–2.5).[45] In secondary analysis of data from a randomized controlled trial, it has been observed that in the low dependence group 2 mg lozenge did not have consistently significant effects on the withdrawal symptoms of emotional distress, but led to significant reductions in craving versus placebo. In the high dependence group (TTFC< 30 minutes), the 4 mg lozenge was associated with significant reductions versus placebo in emotional distress symptoms and craving.[46] The 4 mg nicotine lozenge and 4 mg nicotine gum have comparable safety profiles in patients with heart disease, hypertension not controlled by medication and/or diabetes mellitus.[47]

Patients with TTFC < 30 minutes of waking should use the 4-mg strength lozenge, and others should use the 2-mg strength lozenge. The success rates of the therapy are more if the patients use the lozenge on a fixed schedule rather than as needed. During the initial 6 weeks of therapy, 1 lozenge every 1 to 2 hours while awake.[1] Patients can use additional lozenges (up to 5 lozenges in 6 hours or a maximum of 20 lozenges per day) if cravings occur between scheduled doses. The lozenge should be allowed to dissolve slowly in the mouth; when nicotine is released from the polacrilin resin, a warm, tingling sensation may be experienced. The lozenge should be occasionally rotated to different areas of the mouth to reduce the potential for mucosal irritation. When used correctly, the lozenge dissolves within 30 minutes. The effectiveness of the nicotine lozenge may be reduced by acidic beverages such as coffee, juices, wine, or soft drinks.

ADVERSE EFFECTS

The chewing or swallowing of the lozenge increases the incidence of gastrointestinal-related side effects. The most common adverse effects include nausea, hiccups, cough, dyspepsia, headache, and flatulence. Patients who use more than one lozenge at a time or continuously use one lozenge after another, or chew or swallow the lozenge are more likely to experience dyspepsia or hiccups.

Chapter 7

NICOTINE NASAL SPRAY

The nicotine nasal spray, available as prescription only drug, is another first line medication for treating tobacco use.[1] The nicotine nasal spray is an aqueous solution of nicotine available in a metered-spray pump for administration to the nasal mucosa. The nasal spray was designed to deliver doses of nicotine to the smoker more rapidly than other NRTs. The device is a multidose bottle with pump and each actuation delivers a metered 50-mcL spray containing 0.5 mg of nicotine.

The dose of nicotine (1 mg) is administered as two sprays, one (0.5 mg spray) in each nostril. Following administration of 2 sprays approximately 53%±16% (mean ±SD) enters the systemic circulation.[48] The peak venous nicotine concentrations are achieved within 11 to 18 minutes after administration. (Figure 1) The apparent absorption half-life of nicotine is approximately 3 minutes. There is a wide variation among subjects in their plasma nicotine concentrations from the spray.[48] C_{max} with nicotine nasal spray (2 sprays) is 9±3 ng/ml.

Use of the nicotine nasal spray more than doubles long-term (>6 months) abstinence rates when compared to placebo.[28] A study by Hurt et al suggests that a 1 mg dose of nicotine nasal spray can relieve spontaneous nicotine withdrawal symptoms, including craving, more rapidly than a single dose of 4 mg nicotine gum.[49]

The recommended initial regimen is one to two doses every hour while awake for 6 to 8 weeks and this may be increased as needed. The minimum and maximum recommended doses are 8 doses/day and 5 doses/hour or 40 mg/day respectively. (Table 1) The less frequent administration may be less effective. After 6 to 8 weeks, the dose should be gradually decreased over an additional 4 to 6 weeks.[1]

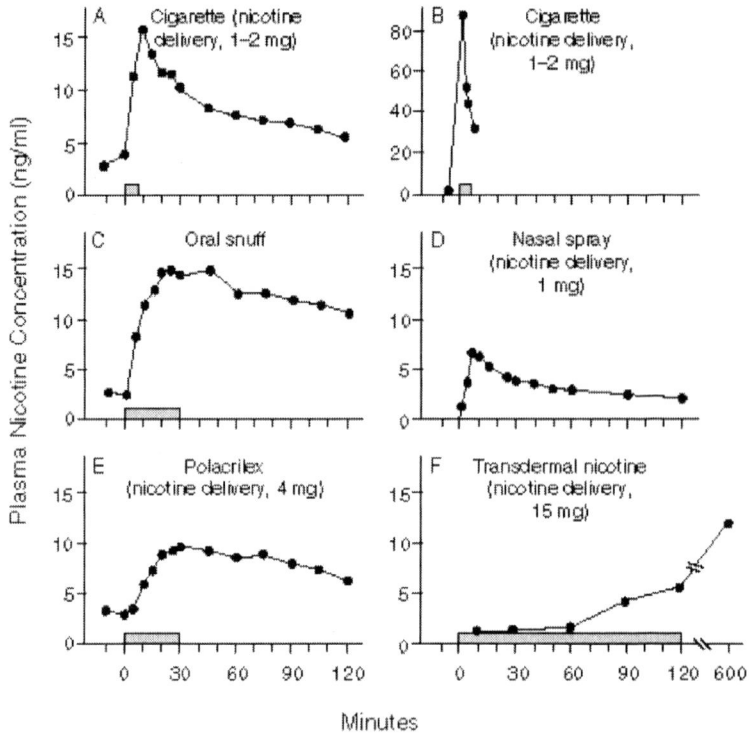

The shaded bar in each panel indicates the period of nicotine delivery. The amount of nicotine delivered from the subjects' standard cigarettes was assumed to be 1 to 2 mg. The data on oral snuff were obtained in 10 subjects after each used 2.5 g of commercially available moist snuff with no nicotine dose specified.[29] All plasma nicotine values are based on samples of venous blood, except those in Panel B, which are based on arterial blood collected in one subject while he smoked a cigarette (data replotted from Henningfield et al.[30]). The data on transdermal nicotine (11 subjects) are replotted from Benowitz[31]; the data in panel A on cigarettes (10 subjects) and on nicotine polacrilex (10 subjects) are from Benowitz et al.[29]; and the data on nasal spray (8 subjects) are from Johansson et al.[32]

Figure 1. Plasma Nicotine concentrations before and after the administration of a single dose of nicotine in several forms. Reprinted with permission from Henningfield JE. Nicotine Medications for smoking Cessation. *New J. Engl. Med.* 1995;333:1196-1203.[25]

ADVERSE EFFECTS

The commonly reported adverse effects with the nicotine nasal spray include nasal and throat irritation (hot peppery sensation), sneezing, coughing, watery eyes, and rhinorrhea. The nicotine nasal spray has a dependence potential intermediate between tobacco products and other NRT products. About 15% to 20% of patients continue to use the nicotine nasal spray for longer periods than recommended (6–12 months), and 5% use the spray at higher doses than recommended.[26] Individuals with chronic nasal disorders (e.g. rhinitis, polyps, sinusitis) or severe reactive airway disease should not use the nicotine nasal spray because of its irritant effects. Although nicotine nasal spray causes substantial irritant side effects during the first few days of use, these adverse effects decrease significantly within the first week.[50]

Chapter 8

NICOTINE INHALER

Nicotine inhaler, a prescription only drug is another first-line medication available for smoking cessation.[1] The inhaler consists of a mouthpiece and a plastic cartridge containing nicotine. The nicotine inhaler treats the complexity of smoking through weaning both from the drug and from the sensory/ritual components associated with smoking. The inhaler is 'puffed' but not lit and there is considerable 'puffing' required to achieve slower rising and lower nicotine concentrations. These factors allow it to be used as a nicotine reduction treatment.[51]

The nicotine inhaler is not a true inhaler as most of the nicotine released from the inhaler is deposited in the mouth. Only a fraction of the dose released, less than 5%, reaches the lower respiratory tract. Each inhaler cartridge contains 10 mg nicotine, of which 4 mg can be delivered and 2 mg is absorbed.[52] Peak plasma concentrations are reached within 15 minutes of the end of inhalation. Absorption of nicotine through the buccal mucosa is relatively slow. This is different from the higher levels and rapid rise followed by the decline in nicotine arterial plasma concentrations seen with cigarette smoking. After use of the single inhaler the arterial nicotine concentrations rise slowly to an average of 6 ng/mL in contrast to those seen with a cigarette, which increase rapidly and reach a mean C_{max} of approximately 49 ng/mL within 5 minutes.[53] Acidic beverages interfere with the buccal absorption of nicotine. The amount of nicotine absorbed from the inhaler is temperature-dependent, with higher ambient air temperatures delivering larger amounts of nicotine and lower temperatures delivering smaller amounts.[54]

In a double blind randomized trial the nicotine inhaler was significantly superior to placebo in achieving reduction in daily cigarette consumption by at least 50% after 4 months, compared with baseline (18% vs 8%, p = .004). Active treatment promoted smoking cessation: 8% of subjects in the nicotine group and 1% in the placebo group were abstinent at 15th month. [55]

A dose from the inhaler consists of a puff or inhalation. Each cartridge delivers a total of 4 mg of nicotine over 80 inhalations. Recommended dosage is 6-16 cartridges /day; continued for upto 6 months.[1] (Table 1) However, the dose should be tapered in final 6-12 weeks of treatment. Till now there are no trials showing the benefits of using nicotine inhaler for more than 6 months.

ADVERSE EFFECTS

The adverse effects include local irritation in the mouth and throat, coughing and rhinitis. These are generally mild and their frequency declines with continued use.[1] The abuse potential with inhaler is less as there is slower absorption, smaller fluctuations in blood levels and low levels of nicotine in serum.

Chapter 9

STATUS AND NEWER RECOMMENDATIONS FOR NRT

Although many formulations are available for nicotine delivery, yet none of them has individually led to a miraculous change in the scenario of smoking in the world. There is a need to improve the regimens and the pharmacokinetic features of the available formulations.

NRT can help in Tobacco Harm Reduction (THR) by various ways. NRT can reduce the relapse rates if they are given for prolonged periods i.e. for more than the specified period. There have been varied results about the benefit of extended therapy. Medioni et al[56] report from a meta-analysis that if NRT had been continued, around 50% of relapses could have been prevented. They conclude that the protective effect of NRT against relapse slowly decreases as a function of time and after stopping NRT, the risk of relapse increases. It may be more beneficial not to stop NRT after the usual 3-6 month treatment period but to use NRT for longer periods of time.[56] Another multicentre, randomized, double-blind placebo-controlled trial reported that a higher than standard dose of nicotine patch was associated with an increase in the long-term success in smoking cessation but continuation of treatment beyond 8-12 weeks did not increase the success rates.[57] A recent parallel, randomized, placebo-controlled trial has shown that transdermal nicotine for 24 weeks increased biochemically confirmed point-prevalence abstinence and continuous abstinence at week 24, reduced the risk for smoking lapses, and increased the likelihood of recovery to abstinence after a lapse compared with 8 weeks of transdermal nicotine therapy.[58] The use of NRT after a lapse to prevent progression can be another effective strategy, as data has shown that after even a single limited exposure to smoking (lapse), the probability of relapse is very high. [59] But, the current labeling implies that smokers should stop using NRT if they start smoking. In some cases NRT can be given for longer periods, even indefinitely to prevent relapse to smoking.[60] Although nicotine is not entirely without risk, nicotine maintenance is clearly safer than cigarette smoke delivered nicotine. In some cases the mainstay of treatment should be reduction in smoking rather than quitting. The use of NRT along with reduced smoking can again decrease the exposure to the toxins usually inhaled with smoking.

NEW FORMULATIONS OF NRT

Sublingual Tablet

A nicotine sublingual tablet is available in some European countries, but not yet approved by FDA for use in US. The levels of nicotine achieved with 2 mg sublingual tablet and 2 mg nicotine gum are similar.[61]

Oral Nicotine

Oral nicotine has not been a route of administration because of high first pass metabolism of nicotine and high incidence of adverse effects like gastrointestinal disturbance. Two products have been proposed for oral delivery: the *straw* and the *nicotine drops*. The straw is a single–use plastic straw containing small beads of nicotine. When a smoker drinks a beverage through the straw, the nicotine beads are swallowed.[62] Similarly the nicotine drops can be used by putting the drops of the nicotine solution in the beverage.[63] Both the delivery systems are being tried.

Pulmonary Delivered Nicotine

A true pulmonary inhaler, unlike the currently available nicotine inhaler (which actually delivers nicotine into the mouth for buccal absorption) would deliver nicotine to the lung in a manner more comparable to cigarette smoking. There are various challenges involved in the development of nicotine inhaler. The nicotine molecules should be condensed to particles of approximately 1 micron median diameter to enable inhalation into the pulmonary alveoli. Another barrier for the development, is its potential for abuse and the regulatory implications that would follow from a system that delivers pulmonary nicotine at levels comparable to that delivered by a cigarette.[24]

PROPOSED METHODS TO INCREASE THE EFFICACY OF NRT

Increasing the Dose

None of the various clinical trials comparing the efficacy and safety of standard and higher dose of nicotine patch have given any conclusive results. As mentioned in the benefits of extended trial, one trial demonstrated that a higher than standard dose of nicotine patch was associated with a modest benefit.[57] Jorenby et al observed that there does not appear to be any general, sustained benefit of initiating transdermal nicotine therapy with a 44-mg patch dose or of providing intense adjuvant smoking cessation treatment. The two doses and all adjuvant treatments produced equivalent effects at the 26-week follow-up, and the higher patch dose produced more adverse effects.[64] On the other hand, another study demonstrated that high-dose transdermal nicotine has low acute toxicity if dosed appropriately and that transdermal nicotine suppresses nicotine and carbon monoxide intake during ad libitum cigarette smoking in smokers who were not trying to quit.[65] So, till now, the standard doses are giving the optimal results, but may be with more large multicentre trials, different results may come up.

Increasing the Delivery Speed

A rapid release gum has been formulated to provide biphasic nicotine delivery. In the initial phase there is accelerated delivery to promote rapid craving relief and then leveling off to avoid overdosing. Niaura et al.[66] compared this rapid-release gum to the current gum formulation for rapid craving relief following a provocative stimulus. The rapid-release gum achieved faster and more complete craving relief, differentiating itself from current nicotine gum within the first 3 minutes of use. The use of such a product to provide rapid craving relief when a rescue medication is needed can forestall relapse and thus enhance clinical efficacy. This new technology for rapid nicotine delivery via the transmucosal route merits further study in cessation efficacy trials.

Presently, comparison of different NRTs in meta-analysis and direct comparative studies have concluded that the nicotine gum, patch, nasal spray and the inhaler treatments appear to be equally efficacious.[67-69]

Chapter 10

BUPROPION

Bupropion, originally marketed for the treatment of depression was the first potent non-nicotine pharmacological treatment approved for smoking cessation.[1] Bupropion is chemically unrelated to tricyclic antidepressants or selective serotonin reuptake inhibitors (SSRIs). Like the NRT products, Bupropion SR (150 mg) has been endorsed by the US Clinical Practice Guidelines as a first line therapy.[1] Bupropion SR (150 mg) is available as a prescription drug only. The immediate release formulation is used in the management of depression.

Smoking and depression are highly associated, as both are influenced by dopamine levels.[70,71] The precise mechanism of action of bupropion as a smoking cessation aid is not clear. It is hypothesized that the mechanism involves both dopaminergic and noradrenergic activity. Bupropion, at therapeutic doses can bind to striatal dopamine transporters (approx. 20% occupancy) and potentially prevent dopamine uptake and thus decrease the negative withdrawal symptoms.[72] Bupropion also reduces the firing rates of noradrenergic neurons in the locus coeruleus which contain neuronal projections to the hippocampus.[73] Bupropion also interacts with nicotinic receptors. As a noncompetitive antagonist of these receptors, bupropion may attenuate the rewarding effects of nicotine.[74,75] Thus, bupropion helps in smoking cessation by decreasing cravings and alleviating withdrawal symptoms in abstinent smokers.

Bupropion is extensively metabolized in humans with less than 1% excreted unchanged in urine. Hydroxybupropion, threohydrobupropion and erythrohydrobupropion are the active biotransformation products in plasma. It has been seen that smoking and gender does not affect the pharmacokinetic parameters of bupropion. In a comparative analysis of the effect of smoking on pharmacokinetics of bupropion it was seen that there was no significant difference in $AUC_{0-\infty}$, mean C_{max}, T_{max} and $t_{½}$ values between the healthy smokers and non-smokers. It was also seen that for sustained release (SR) preparation the T_{max} values of bupropion and its metabolites were greater and the C_{max} values of bupropion and its metabolites were lower as compared to the immediate release (IR) preparation.[76]

In large number of comparative studies, Bupropion SR has been proved to be more efficacious than placebo in improving smoking cessation.[77-81] In some controlled trials, head to head comparisons among the various available drugs have also been done. In a direct comparison of sustained release Bupropion and transdermal nicotine patch, significantly higher abstinence was found with combination therapy (Bupropion SR + Transdermal Nicotine Patch) (35.5%) as compared to Bupropion SR alone (30.3%) and with transdermal nicotine alone (16.4%) at 12 months.[82]

The recommended and maximum dose of Bupropion SR is 300 mg/day, given as 150 mg twice daily.[1]

ADVERSE EFFECTS

The most serious adverse effect is seizure, which affects an estimated 1 in 1000 users. More common side effects include dry mouth, insomnia, skin rash, pruritis and hypersensitivity. Rarely there may be a reaction resembling serum sickness. Serious neuropsychiatric symptoms have been reported in post marketing surveillances. These include changes in mood (including depression and mania), psychosis, hallucinations, paranoia, delusions, homicidal ideation, hostility, agitation, aggression, anxiety, and panic, as well as suicidal ideation, suicide attempt, and completed suicide. Some reported cases have been complicated by the symptoms of nicotine withdrawal in patients who stopped smoking. Depressed mood may be a symptom of nicotine withdrawal. Depression, rarely including suicidal ideation, has been reported in smokers undergoing a smoking cessation attempt. In July, 2009 US FDA asked the manufacturers to add a boxed warning on the prescribing information of Bupropion SR (Zyban).[83] Bupropion is contraindicated in patients with current or past epilepsy, or history of anorexia nervosa and bulimia, severe hepatic necrosis or bipolar disease.[84]

Chapter 11

VARENICLINE

Varenicline is a partial agonist of the $\alpha_4\beta_2$ nicotinic cholinergic receptor. In May 2006, Varenicline was approved by FDA for smoking cessation in cigarette smokers ages 18 and above.[85] The structure of varenicline is based on the alkaloid extract cytisine, which was earlier used in the European countries for smoking cessation.[86] Varenicline has a dual action as it blocks nicotine from binding to the receptor (antagonist action) and partially stimulates (agonist action) receptor mediated activity, leading to the release of dopamine, which reduces cravings and nicotine withdrawal symptoms.[87] Partial agonists have been shown to be less susceptible to abuse in comparison to the full agonists.[88,89]

Varenicline is completely absorbed orally and not affected by food. Steady state is reached within four days of administration. The time to reach maximum concentration is three to four hours. Varenicline exhibits linear kinetics. Varenicline has low protein binding (≤20%) and is not metabolized, unlike nicotine, which undergoes hepatic metabolism by CYP2A6. Most of the drug (92%) is excreted unchanged in the urine via glomerular filtration and active tubular secretion via organic cation transporters. Varenicline has a half-life of 24 hours.[90] Mild renal failure does not affect varenicline's area under the concentration-time curve (AUC), though moderate to severe renal failure does increase the AUC about 1.5-2-fold. However, this increase in the AUC is not thought to be clinically significant.[91]

In various phase II and phase III trials, varenicline has been compared with placebo, Bupropion SR and NRT. In two phase III trials, varenicline 1 mg BID was shown to be more efficacious than placebo and Bupropion SR 150 mg BID. The continence abstinence rates at week 12 were ≈44% for Varenicline versus ≈30% for Bupropion SR and ≈18% for placebo.[92,93]

An additional 12 weeks of varenicline has been shown to be effective in maintaining smoking abstinence in smokers who had stopped smoking after 12 weeks of open label varenicline treatment.[94] In an interventinal review Cahill et al[95] concluded that varenicline increased the chances of successful long-term smoking cessation by between two- and three fold compared with pharmacologically unassisted quit attempts; more people quit successfully with varenicline than with bupropion; the effectiveness of varenicline as an aid to relapse prevention has not been clearly established.

Varenicline should be initiated at a dose of 0.5 mg once daily for the first three days, followed by 0.5 mg twice daily for the next four days and then 1 mg twice daily for the remainder of the treatment period. Length of treatment should be at least 12 weeks and can be extended for an additional 12 weeks. Longer treatments can be recommended for abstinent smokers who are concerned about smoking relapse.[10,85]

ADVERSE EVENTS

Mild to moderate nausea is the most frequent adverse effect of varenicline. Vivid dreams were the next common adverse event. In February 2008, the FDA added a warning regarding its use. It noted that depressed mood, agitation, changes in behavior, suicidal ideation and suicide have been reported in patients attempting to quit smoking while using varenicline.[96] The FDA recommends that patients should tell their health care provider about any history of psychiatric illness prior to starting medication and clinicians should monitor patients for change in mood and behavior while on varenicline.[1] Cahill et al[97] have reported that much of the reported behavioral and mood changes may be associated with nicotine withdrawal, although some effects occurred in people who continued to smoke while taking the medication. Gunnell D et al[98] concluded that there is no clear evidence of an increased risk of self harm, suicidal thoughts, or depression in people prescribed varenicline compared with those prescribed other smoking cessation products. But, in view of increasing concerns about the possible increased risk of suicide associated with these drugs, further investigation of their effect on suicide risk is required in other databases and through secondary analysis of all adverse events reporting in relevant clinical trials. In view of this, patients and their caregivers should be alerted about the need to monitor for neuropsychiatric symptoms including changes in behavior.

Chapter 12

CLONIDINE

Clonidine an α_2 adrenergic receptor agonist which was initially used for the treatment of hypertension, was later found to diminish both opiate and alcohol withdrawal syndrome.[68,72] Glassman and colleagues demonstrated the efficacy of Clonidine for reducing nicotine craving and withdrawal symptoms in heavy cigarette smokers.[99]

Presently, Clonidine is not approved by FDA for smoking cessation, but it has been endorsed as second line medication for treating tobacco use by the US Clincal Practice Guidelines.[1] Various meta-analyses done in the last two decades have shown varied results. In the meta-analysis by Covey and Glassman[100], the combined odds ratios for success indicated that smokers treated with clonidine were significantly more likely to quit smoking than those treated with placebo. Gourlay and Benowitz[101] observed high frequency of adverse effects with a significantly higher long term quit rate with clonidine therapy. They concluded that clonidine may be helpful for smoking cessation in the short term, its benefit may be limited to smokers who experience high levels of agitation and anxiety when they stop smoking. A recent Cochrane analysis reviewed the efficacy of clonidine for smoking cessation from six studies and found that clonidine treatment was associated with increased smoking cessation [pooled odds ratio of 1.89 (95% CI:1.30-2.74)]; however when analyzed separately only one study showed significant improvement in smoking cessation.[102] Some evidence also suggests that clonidine is more effective in women than men.[103,104] Clonidine should be started shortly before (upto 3 days) or on the quit date.[1] Clonidine is available both as tablets and trandermal patches.

ADVERSE EFFECTS

The adverse effects associated with clonidine use such as drowsiness, fatigue and dry mouth, postural hypotension limit its use. Discontinuation should be slow to avoid rebound hypertension.

Chapter 13

NORTRIPTYLINE

Of the antidepressants tested for efficacy in smoking cessation, tricyclic antidepressants have shown promising results. Nortriptyline has been considered appropriate as a second line medication for treating tobacco use.[1] Nortriptyline inhibits both serotonin and noradrenaline reuptake for the treatment of depression. Nortriptyline has been studied for smoking cessation in monotherapy[105,106] and combination therapy.[107] Various clinical trials have demonstrated the potential efficacy of nortriptyline for smoking cessation in smokers without history of major depression[105] or with such history.[106] The smoking cessation rates achieved with nortriptyline appear to be comparable to those achieved with Bupropion SR [pooled odds ratios:2:1(1.5-3.1) versus 2.0 (1.7-3.4)].[108]

According to US Public Health Service Guidelines 2008[1], smoking cessation trials have initiated treatment at a dose of 25 mg/day, increasing gradually to a target dose of 75-100 mg/day. Duration of treatment in the trials has been 12 weeks although clinicians may extend the treatment upto 6 months.[1] It is recommended that the therapy should be initiated 10-28 days before the quit date so that steady state levels of nortriptyline can be reached. Nortriptyline should not be abruptly discontinued.

ADVERSE EFFECTS

Most common side effects are sedation, dry mouth (64-78%), blurred vision (16%), urinary retention, lightheadedness (49%) and shaky hands.[1] The mental and/or physical abilities may be impaired. As there is a risk of arrhythmias and impairment of myocardial contractility, it should be used with caution in patients with cardiovascular disease.[1] Nortriptyline should not be co-administered with MAO inhibitors.

NEWER FORMULATIONS FOR NORTRIYPTYLINE

Transdermal patches[109] and iontophoresis[110] formulations for nortriptyline are under investigations.

Chapter 14

NICOTINIC OR NON-NICOTINIC THERAPIES UNDER INVESTIGATION

NICOTINE VACCINES

One novel approach undergoing investigation is immunization against nicotine. Vaccination was first suggested as a strategy for treating drug dependence more than 30 years ago.[111] In drug dependence, vaccines are intended to elicit the production of antibodies which will bind the drug in question and alter its pharmacokinetics in a manner that is therapeutically helpful. A vaccine against nicotine induces nicotine specific antibodies (NicAb) that can bind nicotine molecules in plasma before the drug reaches the neural receptors which are responsible for producing effects normally associated with smoking. The antibodies themselves are too large to cross the blood-brain barrier, so that administered nicotine which becomes bound to antibody is also excluded from the brain. It has been seen that immunization with a nicotine vaccine prevented the nicotine-induced increase in dopamine release in the shell of the Nucleus Accumbens.[112]

All three of the current nicotine conjugate vaccines in clinical trials (Nic-VAX, NicQb and TIA-NIC) were well tolerated in phase I trials with no evidence of untoward cross reactivity with endogenous neurotransmitters or other signaling molecules. Nic-VAX is a recombinant *Pseudomonas aeruginosa* exoprotein A conjugate vaccine.[113] CYT002-NicQb is based on the virus-like particle formed by the recombination coat protein of the bacteriophage Qb.[114] TA-NIC is an immunotherapeutic vaccine. Results of phase I and II have reported no unexpected adverse events and its efficacy as compared to placebo.[115]

Enhanced smoking cessation rates have been reported in clinical trials of nicotine vaccines, but they are confined to those subjects with the highest serum antobody concentrations.[113,116] Two limitations of vaccination are apparent from the trials. First, the mean serum NicAb concentrations are lower than those reported in rats and mice.[117,118] Second, there is a substantial variability (upto a 30 fold range) in these concentrations. There is a need to develop strategies to reliably produce high serum antibody concentrations in response to nicotine vaccines so as to maximize their efficacy. Passive immunization with nicotine specific monoclonal antibodies is being studied in animals.[119] Comparative analysis of vaccination vs passive immunization with nicotine antibodies vs combination of active and passive immunization is being studied. The advantage of combination therapy is the rapid production of uniformly high concentrations of NicAb concentrations. The main disadvantage of passive immunization is its cost; as it is expensive than active immunization with vaccines.

Vaccination is not likely to duplicate or replace the existing medications. It will not reduce the severity of tobacco withdrawal as is done by most of the medications. Vaccination will help in blunting the rewarding effects of nicotine, something which is not the mechanism of action of the currently available drugs. Vaccination will also be better suited for relapse prevention, in which the goal is to block the priming effect of few cigarettes, than for smoking cessation independently.

Chapter 15

RIMONABANT

In the last decade of the twentieth century, the possible involvement of endocannabinoid system in drug dependence was suggested.[120,121] Cannabinoids (CBs) are a group of chemical compounds that act as ligands to G-protein coupled cannabinoid receptors. The cannabinoids can be herbal, endogenous or synthetic. The endogenous include N-arachidonylethanolamine (AEA) and 2-arachidonoyl glycerol (2-AG). Till now, two CB receptors (CB1 and CB2) have been identified. Gonzalez et al found that chronic nicotine exposure increased AEA levels in the limbic forebrain and brainstem but decreased levels in the hippocampus, striatum. [122]

Rimonabant, a CB antagonist was tested in three trials for its role in smoking cessation. In STRATUS-US trial[123], significantly higher number of patients receiving 20 mg rimonabant remained abstinent compared with those who were on 5 mg (15.6% and 16.1% placebo). In contrast, another study (STRATUS-Europe)[124] with same duration of treatment and follow-up period, found no significant increase in smoking cessation for either treatment dose groups (5 and 20 mg) compared to placebo group (24%, 25% and 20% respectively). The third study (STRATUS-Worldwide)[124] was maintenance of abstinence trial examining one year of treatment outcomes. Patients receiving 20 mg rimonabant ($\approx$ 42%) remained smoke free for the entire year compared to patients receiving placebo treatment ($\approx$ 32 %). However, in late 2008, Sanofi-aventis[125], the company carrying on the trials with Rimonabant stopped the further research after repeated efforts of various organizations. It was reported that rimonabant leads to severe depression and increases the suicidal tendencies.

Chapter 16

MECAMYLAMINE

Mecamylamine, a nicotinic antagonist, was used as an antihypertensive till 1996. It blocks the peripheral and CNS effects of nicotine. Mecamylamine was one of the first medications studied for smoking cessation treatment. Unfortunately, intolerable side–effects including constipation, drowsiness and dry mouth caused by the high doses employed (mean 26.7 mg/day) outweighed the drug's beneficial effects on smoking cessation.[126] However, Rose et al[127] found that a very low dose of mecamylamine (2.5 mg/day), which was well tolerated, also reduced the subjective desire to smoke. Later, efficacy of low doses of mecamylamine plus nicotine was studied as investigators thought that nicotine and mecamylamine would work in concert to attenuate the rewarding effects of cigarette smoking and suppress the withdrawal symptoms. At low doses, mecamylamine is effective at blocking the rewarding effects of nicotine and enhancing short-term cessation in conjunction with nicotine patch. [128,129] Moreover, the low doses do not precipitate withdrawal.[130] Mecamylamine has little effect on the clearance of co-administered nicotine, but reduces the volume of distribution of nicotine. In a trial investigating gender effects in the treatment of smoking cessation Rose et al[131] found that administration of mecamylamine prior to quitting smoking may be necessary to extinguish the influence of environmental cues previously reinforced by smoking. Moreover, they found that abstinence rates were much higher for women receiving mecamylamine than for men.[131] Mecamylamine may decrease the potential adverse cardiovascular effects of co-administered nicotine.[132] Additional studies are required to ascertain the long term effectiveness of mecamylamine in smoking cessation.

Chapter 17

INHIBITORS OF NICOTINE METABOLISM

Nicotine elimination is a major factor in determining the number of cigarettes smoked. So reduction in elimination of nicotine can be a novel strategy for smoking cessation. In humans, approximately 70-80% of nicotine is metabolised to cotinine.[133] The majority of this metabolic conversion is catalyzed by the genetically polymorphic CYP2A6 enzyme.[134] Any change in the amount or function of this enzyme will significantly affect plasma nicotine level during smoking and during NRT treatment and thus may alter smoking behaviors and the efficacy of NRT products.

Genetic variations in the CYP2A6 allele have been shown to strongly affect both nicotine pharmacokinetics as well as smoking behavior. For instance, CYP2A6*4 is a gene deletion variant where no enzyme is produced; individuals with 2 alleles of this variant have impaired nicotine metabolism forming very low levels of cotinine.[135,136] In terms of smoking behaviors, slower metabolizers (individuals with ≤50% in nicotine metabolism activity) consume fewer cigarettes per day (as indicated by self-report and lower carbon-monoxide levels), and are at a lower risk for being dependent smokers.[137-139] Based on this, it was hypothesized that smoking can be reduced by mimicking the defects in CYP2A6 enzyme. And the long term behavioral effects of these inhibitors may be predicted based on available pharmacogenetic and behavioral studies.

CYP2A6 inhibitors Methoxsalen and Tranylcypromine have been studied in experimental settings. Concurrent use of these with NRT products may enhance smoking cessation. It has been seen that with Methoxsalen plus nicotine gum the mean plasma nicotine levels are significantly higher compared to placebo plus nicotine gum.[140] Studies of CYP2A6 inhibition with oral nicotine have also shown increased levels of mean plasma nicotine levels and decreased desire of smokers to smoke.[141] Currently these inhibitors are undergoing trials. These can be helpful in harm reduction in future.

Chapter 18

OPIOID ANTAGONISTS

As discussed in the mechanism of dependence, many other neurotransmitters and modulators including endogenous opioid peptides are involved in nicotine dependence. Studies involving Naloxone and Naltrexone have given confusing results. Cochrane analysis of opioid antagonists for their role in smoking cessation in 2001[142] and 2006[143] have shown that all four trials of naltrexone failed to detect a significant difference in quit rates between naltrexone and placebo. In a pooled analysis there was no significant effect of naltrexone on long-term abstinence, and confidence intervals were wide (odds ratio 1.26, 95% confidence interval 0.80 to 2.01). Also, no trials of naloxone or buprenorphine reported long-term follow up. Nalmefene, another opioid antagonist currently marketed in the US as an injectable formulation, is also undergoing evaluation for tobacco dependence program.[144]

Chapter 19

ANTIDEPRESSANTS

Other than Bupropion and Nortriptyline, which are approved as first line and second line agents for smoking cessation therapy respectively, other antidepressants have demonstrated only modest results. Venlafaxine, a selective serotonin reuptake inhibitor (SSRI) and an atypical antidepressant has shown only limited efficacy among light smokers as a tobacco dependence treatment.[145] Fluoxetine, another SSRI has minimal effect on norepinephrine and dopamine reuptake. Results of a large, randomized, double-blind, placebo-controlled, multi-centre, clinical trial reveal that among heavy smokers, 30 mg/day and 60 mg/day doses of fluoxetine significantly enhance short-term abstinence rates compared with placebo.[146] Three studies have shown that among abstinent smokers, there is less weight gain associated with smoking cessation while using fluoxetine relative to placebo.[147-149] Paroxetine has not shown significant results in studies comparing nicotine trandermal patch and placebo alongwith.[150] Moclobemide, a monoamine amine oxidase (MAO) inhibitor increases synaptic concentrations of noradrenaline, serotonin and dopamine. In a randomized double-blind, parallel-group, placebo-controlled, single-centre study, heavy smokers were treated with moclobemide 400 mg/day beginning 1 week prior to their quit date and thereafter for 2 months, reducing to 200 mg/day for another month. In contrast to self-administered abstinence, verified abstinence did not differ significantly between treatment conditions at 6 months or 1 year follow-up.[151] Taken together, these findings show that fluoxetine and other SSRI medications may be helpful in smokers concerned about weight gain.

Chapter 20

GABAERGIC AGENTS

It is hypothesized that the agents that affect GABA neurotransmission may decrease the reinforcing properties of nicotine. Dopaminergic neurons projecting from the ventral tegmental area (VTA) to the nucleus accumbens receive descending GABAergic input from the ventral pallidum and the nucleus accumbens.[152] Dopaminergic tone in the VTA and nucleus accumbens is inhibited by these GABAergic neurons. At the VTA, inhibition of dopaminergic activity involves GABAergic inhibitory afferents to dopaminergic ventral tegmental neurons and interneurons within the VTA.[153,154] Baclofen, a selective $GABA_B$ agonist has shown decrease in nicotine self-administraion in rats.[155,156] Tiagabine has also been studied in smokers.[157] Till now, there has been relatively little study of these medications in clinical trials. However, more data can help in reaching at some conclusion about the use of these agents in smoking cessation.

Chapter 21

DRUG THERAPY IN PREGNANT FEMALES

Pregnant women who continue to smoke expose their developing fetus to a wide range of risks. Assisting these patients to stop smoking can be an important intervention for the health of the baby and the mother. The management of pregnant smokers can be challenging, due to the potential risks of pharmacotherapy. At present the guidelines do not recommend any particular group of drugs for smoking cessation in pregnant women.

It is known that nicotine through its actions on nicotinic cholinergic receptors, elicits abnormalities of neural cell proliferation and differentiation, promotes apoptosis and produces deficits in the number of neural cells and in synaptic function. The effects eventually compromise multiple neurotransmitter systems because of the widespread regulatory role of cholinergic neurotransmission. Importantly, the long-term alterations include effects on reward systems that reinforce the subsequent susceptibility to nicotine addiction in later life.[158] It has been reported in animal studies that maternal nicotine exposure induces a persistent inhibition of glycolysis and a drastically increased AMP level. These metabolic changes are thought to contribute to the faster aging of the lungs of the offspring of mothers that are exposed to nicotine via the placenta and mother's milk. The lungs of these animals are more susceptible to damage as shown by the gradual deterioration of the lung parenchyma.[159] The use of NRT or varenicline is not approved in pregnant women as yet. Various trials reported so far have not led to any conclusive result.[1]

Chapter 22

CRITICAL ISSUES OF PHARMACOTHERAPY

Status of the currently available drugs: According to the findings of an updated meta-analysis of smoking cessation pharmacotherapy by Canadian investigators, all 7 first line therapies are superior to placebo, and the highest point estimate of the 7 first-line therapies was observed for varenicline (OR, 2.55;95%CI,1.99-3.24).[160]

Combination therapy: Trials evaluating the combination therapy have shown better results as compared to monotherapy e.g. combination of transdermal nicotine patch and nortriptyline[161], combination of nicotine patch and the lozenge[162,163], Bupropion SR + lozenge (odds ratio, 0.46-0.56)[162], combination of varenicline and bupropion[164] with few exceptions.[165]

Extended duration of therapy: Various trials have shown that drugs when given for a longer period lead to better abstinence rates.[166]

Changing the target population: More programs are needed to target specific groups like young adults and pregnant females. The young people have both the greatest propensity to quit and the greatest potential benefits from smoking cessation. Presently, tobacco marketers concentrate on recapturing young quitters, while organized smoking cessation programs are primarily used by older smokers.

REFERENCES

[1] Fiore MC, Jaen CR, Baker TB, Bailey WC, Benowitz NL, Curry SJ et al. Treating Tobacco Use and dependence: 2008 Update. Clinical Practice Guideline, Rockville,MD: U.S. Department of Health and Human services. *Public Health Service.* May 2008

[2] WHO report on the Global Tobacco Epidemic, 2008: The MPOWER package. Geneva. *World Health Organisation,* 2008

[3] Centres for Disease Control and Prevention. Annual smoking-attributable mortality, years of potential life lost, and economic costs- United states,1995-1999. Mor*b. Mortal Wkly Rep.* 2002;51:300-303

[4] Mokdad AH, Mark JS, Stroup DF, Gerberding JL. Actual causes of death in the United States, 2000. *JAMA.* 2004;291:1238-1245

[5] Zwar N, Richmond R, Borland R, Peters M, Stillman S, Litt J et al. Smoking cessation pharmacotherapy: an update for health professionals. Melbourne: The Royal Australian College of General Practitioners, 2007

[6] Centres for Disease Control and Prevention. Smoking-attributable mortality, years of potential life lost, and productivity losses- United States, 2000-2004. *MMWR Morb. Mortal Wkly Rep.* 2008;57:1226-28

[7] Liu BQ, Peto R, Chen ZM, Boreham J, Wu YP, Li JY et al Emerging tobacco hazards in China:1 Retrospective proportional mortality study of one million deaths. *BMJ.* 1998;317:1411-22

[8] Gajalakshmi V, Peto R, Kanaka ST, Jha P. Smoking and mortality from tuberculosis and other diseases in India: Retrospective study of 43,000 adult male deaths and 35000 controls. *Lancet.* 2003;362:507-15

[9] Bader P, McDonald P, Selby P. An algorithim for tailoring pharmacotherapy for smoking cessation: results from a Delphi panel of international experts. *Tobacco Control.* 2009;18:34-42

[10] Hurt RD, Ebbert JO, Hays T, Mcfadden DD. Treating Tobacco Dependence in a Medical Setting. *CA Cancer J. Clin.* 2009;59:314-326.
[11] Benowitz NL. Pharmacology of nicotine: addiction and therapeutics. *Annu. Rev. Pharmacol. Toxicol.* 1996;36:597-613.
[12] Henningfield JE, Keenan RM. Nicotine delivery kinetics and abuse liability. *J. Consult. Cin. Psychol.* 1993;61:743-50
[13] Rang HP, Dale MM, Ritter JM, Flower RJ. Other transmitters and modulators. In Rang and Dale's Pharmacology. Eds Dimock K, McGrath S, Cook L. 6th edition. Churchill Livingston Elsevier London. 2007;Pg 492-507.
[14] Grottick AJ, Trube G, Corrigall WA, Huwyler J, Malherbe P, Wyler R et al. Evidence that nicotinic alpha(7) receptors are not involved in the hyperlocomotor and rewarding effects of nicotine. *J. Pharmacol. Exp. Ther.* 2000;294:1112-9
[15] Maskos U, Molles BE, Pons S, Besson M, Guiard BP, Guilloux BP et al. Nicotine reinforcement and cognition restored by targeted expression of nicotinic receptors. *Nature.* 2005;436:103-7.
[16] Picciotto MR, Zoli M, Rimondini R, Lena C, Marubio LM, Pich EM et al. Acetylcholine receptors containing the beta2 subunit are involved in the reinforcing properties of nicotine. *Nature.* 1998;391:173-7
[17] Walters CL, Brown S, Changeux JP, Martin B, Damaj MI. The beta2 but not alpha7 subunit of the nicotinic acetylcholine receptor is required for nicotine-conditioned place preference in mice. *Psychopahrmacology.* (Berl) 2006;184:339-44
[18] Luscher C. Drugs of abuse. In Basic and Clinical Pharmacology. Eds Katzung BG. 10th edition. Singapore 2007,Pg 511- 524
[19] Tomkins DM, Sellers EM. Addiction and the brain: the role of neurotransmitters in the cause and treatment of drug dependence. *CMAJ.* 2001;164:817-21
[20] Nestler FJ. Is there a common molecular pathway for addiction? *Nat. Neurosci.* 2005;8:1445-49
[21] Rang HP, Dale MM, Ritter JM, Flower RJ. Drug addiction, dependence and abuse. In Rang and Dale's Pharmacology. Eds Dimock K, McGrath S, Cook L. 6th Edition. Churchill Livingston Elsevier. London. 2007;Pg 619-637.
[22] Benowitz NL. Pharmacology of Nicotine addiction, Smoking-Induced disease and Therapeutics. *Annu. Rev. Pharmacol. Toxicol.* 2009;49:57-71.

[23] Balfour DJK. The psychobiology of nicotine dependence. *Eur. Respir. Rev.* 2008;17:172-81

[24] Buchhalter AR, Fant RV, Henningfield JE. Novel pharmacological approaches for treating tobacco dependence and withdrawal: Current Status. *Drugs.* 2008;68:1067-1088

[25] Henningfield JE. Nicotine Medications for smoking Cessation. *New J. Engl. Med.* 1995;333:1196-1203

[26] Henningfield JE, Fant RV, Buchhalter AR, Stitzer ML. Pharmacotherapy of Nicotine Dependence. CA *Cancer J. clin.* 2005;55:281-299

[27] Foulds J, Steinberg MB, Williams JM, Ziedonis DM. Developments in pharmacotherapy for tobacco dependence: past, present and future. *Drug Alcohol. Rev.* 2006;25:59-71

[28] Corelli RL, Hudmon KS. Tobacco Use and dependence. In Applied Therapeutics: The Clinical Use of Drugs 9th edition. Eds Koda-Kimble MA, Young LY, Kradjan WA, Guglielmo BJ, Alldredge BK, Corelli Rl, Williams BR. Chapter 85.Wolter Kluwer Lippincott. 2008:85.1-85.30

[29] Benowitz NL, Porchet H, Sheiner L, Jacob P III. Nicotine absorption and cardiovascular effects with smokeless tobacco use: comparison with cigarettes and nicotine gum. *Clin. Pharmacol. Ther.* 1988;44:23-28

[30] Henningfield JE, Stapleton JM, Benowitz NL, Grayson RF, London ED. Higher levels of nicotine in arterial than in venous blood after cigarette smoking. *Drug Alcohol Depend.* 1993;33:23-29

[31] Benowitz NL. Nicotine replacement therapy: what has been accomplished -- can we do better? *Drugs.* 1993;45:157-170

[32] Johansson CJ, Olsson P, Bende M, Carlsson T, Gunnarsson PO. Absolute bioavailability of nicotine applied to different nasal regions. *Eur. J. Clin. Pharmacol.* 1991;41:585-588

[33] Lancaster T, Stead L, Silagy C, Sowden A. Effectiveness of interventions to help people stop smoking: findings from the Cochrane Library. *BMJ.* 2000;321:355-8

[34] Shiffman S, Shadel WG, Niaura R, Khayrallah MA, Jorenby DDE, Ryan CF et al. Efficacy of acute administration of nicotine gum in relief of cue-provoked cigarette craving. Psychopharmacology 2003;166:343-50

[35] Cohen LM, Collins FL, Brt DM. The effect of chewing gum on tobacco withdrawal. *Addict. Behav.* 1997;22:669-773

[36] Sobue S, Sekiguchi K, Kikkawa H, Irie S. Effect of application sites and multiple doses on nicotine pharmacokinetics in healthy male Japanese smokers following application of the transdermal nicotine patch. *J. Clin. Pharmacol.* 2005;45:1391
[37] Fant RV, Henningfield JE, Shiffman S, Strahs KR, Reitberg DP. A pharmacokinetic crossover study to compare the absorption characteristics of three transdermal nicotine patches. *Pharmacol. Biochem. Behav.* 2000;67:479-82
[38] Bur A, Joukhadar C, Klein N, Herkner H, Mitulovic G, Schmid R et al. Effect of exercise on transdermal nicotine release in healthy habitual smokers. *Int. J. Clin. Pharmacol. Ther.* 2005;43:239-43
[39] Shiffman S, Elash CA, Paton SM, Gwaltney CJ, Paty JA, Clark DM et al. Comparative efficacy of 24-hour and 16 hour transdermal nicotine patches for relief of morning craving. *Addiction.* 2000;95:1185-95
[40] Yun HY, Seo JW, Choi JE, Baek IH, Kang W, Kwon KI. Effects of smoking on the pharmacokinetics and pharmacodynamics of a nicotine patch. *Biopharm. Drug Dispos.* 2008;29:521-8
[41] Shiffman S, Ferguson SG. Nicotine patch therapy prior to quitting smoking: a meta-analysis. *Addiction.* 2008;103:557-63
[42] Hajek P, West R, Foulds J, Nilsson F, Burrow S, Meadow A. randomized comparative trial of nicotine polacrilex, a transdermal patch, nasal spray and an inhaler. *Arch. Intern. Med.* 1999;159:2033-38
[43] Choi JH, Dresler CM, Norton MR, Strahs KR. Pharmacokinetics of a nicotine polacrilex lozenge. *Nicotine Tob. Res.* 2003;5:635-44
[44] Shiffman S, Dresler CM, Hajek P, Gilburt SJ, Targett DA, Strahs KR. Efficacy of a nicotine lozenge for smoking cessation. *Arch. Intern. Med.* 2002;162:1267-76
[45] Stead LF, Perera R, Bullen C, Mant D, Lancaster T. Nicotine replacement therapy for smoking cessation. *Cochrane Database of Systemic Reviews. 2008;*CD000146.
[46] Shiffman S. Effect of nicotine lozenges on affective smoking withdrawal symptoms: secondary analysis of a randomized, double-blind, placebo-controlled clinical trial. *Cin. Ther.* 2008;30:1461-75
[47] Marsh HS, Dresler CM, Choi DJ, Targett DA, Gamble ML, Strahs KR. Safety profile of a nicotine lozenge compared with that of nicotine gum in adult smokers with underlying medical conditions: A 12 week, randomized, open-label study. *Clin. Ther.* 2005;27:1571-1567
[48] Pfizer. Nicotrol nasal spray.

http://media.pfizer.com/files/products/uspi_nicotrol.pdf (Last accessed on 3rd May, 2010)

[49] Hurt RD, Offord KP, Crogan IT, Gomez-Dahl LC, Wolter TD, Dale LC, Moyer TP. Temporal effects of nicotine nasal spray and gum on nicotine withdrawal symptoms. *Psychopharmacology.* 1998;140:98-104

[50] Hurt RD, Dale LC, Croghan GA, Croghan IT,Gomez-Dahl LC, Offord KP. Nicotine nasal spray for smoking cessation: pattern of use, side-effects, relief of withdrawal symptoms and cotinine levels. *Mayo Clin. Proc.* 1998;73:118-25

[51] Schneider NG, Olmstead RE, Franzon MA, Lumell E. The nicotine inhaler: clinical pharmacokinetics and comparison with other nicotine treatments. *Clin. Pharmacokinet.* 2001;40:661-84

[52] Molander L, Lunell E, Andersson SB, Kuylenstierna F. Dose released and absolute bioavailability of nicotine from a nicotine vapor inhaler. *Clin. Pharmacol. Ther.* 1996; 59: 394–400

[53] Pfizer. http://media.pfizer.com/files/products/uspi_nicotrol_inhaler.pdf (Last accessed on 28th April,2010)

[54] Lunell E, Molander L, Andersson SB. Temperature dependency of the release and bioavailability of nicotine from a nicotine vapour inhaler; in vitro/ in vivo correlation. *Eur. J. Clin. Pharmacol.* 1997; 52: 495–500

[55] Rennard SI, Glover ED, Leischow S, Daughton DM, Glover PN, Muramoto M et al. Efficacy of a nicotine inhaler in smoking reduction: A double-blind, randomized trial. *Nicotine Tob. Res.* 2006;8:555-64

[56] Medioni J, Berlin I, Mallet A. Increased risk of relapse after stopping nicotine replacement therapies: a mathematical approach. *Addiction.* 2005;100:247-54

[57] Tonnesen P, Paoletti P, Gustavsson G, Russell MA, Saracci R, Gulsvik A et al. Higher dosage nicotine patches increase one year smoking cessation rates: results from the European CEASE trial. Collabrative European Anti-Smoking Evaluation European Respiratory Society. *Eur. Respir. J.* 1999;13:238-246.

[58] Schnoll RA, Patterson F, Wileyto P, Heitjan DF, Shields AE, Asch DA et al. Effectiveness of extended duration of transdermal nicotine therapy. A Randomized Trial. *Ann. Int. Med.* 2010;152:144-151

[59] Baer JS, Kamarck T, Lichtenstein E, Ransom CC, Jr. Prediction of smoking relapse: analysis of temptations and transgressions after initial cessation. *J. Consult. Clin. Psychol.* 1989;57:623-627

[60] Shiffman S, Gitchell JG, Warner KE, Henningfield JE, Pinney JM. Tobacco harm reduction: conceptual structure and nomenclature for analysis and research. *Nicotine Tob. Res.* 2002;4 (Suppl 2):S113-S129

[61] Molander L, Lunell E. Pharmacokinetic investigation of a nicotine sublingual tablet. *Eur. J. Clin. Pharmacol.* 2001;56:813-19

[62] D'Orlando KJ, Fox BS. Tolerability and pharmacokinetics of single and repeated doses of nicotine with The Straw, a novel nicotine replacement product. *Nicotine Tob. Res.* 2004;6:63-70

[63] Westman EC, Tomlin KF, Perkins CE, Rose JE. Oral nicotine solution for smoking cessation: a pilot tolerability study. *Nicotine Tob. Res.* 2001;3:391-6

[64] Jorenby DE, Smith SS, Fiore MC, Hurt RD, Offord KP, Crogan I et al Varying nicotine patch dose and type of smoking cessation counseling. *JAMA.* 1995;274:1347-1352.

[65] Benowitz NL, Zevin S, Jacob PIII. Suppression of nicotine intake during ad libitum cigarette smoking by high-dose transdermal nicotine. *JPET.* 1998;287:958-62

[66] Niaura R, Sayette M, Shiffman S, Glover ED, Nides M, Shelanski M, shadel W et al. Comparative efficacy of rapid-release nicotine gum versus nicotine polacrilex gum in relieving smoking cue-provoked craving. *Addiction.* 2005;100:1720-30

[67] Silagy C, Lancaster T, Stead L, Mant D, Fowler G. Nicotine replacement therapy for smoking cessation. *Cochrane Database system Rev.* 2004;3:CD000146

[68] Covey LS, Sullivan MA, Johnston JA, Glassman AH, Robinson MD, Adams DP. Advances in Non-Nicotine Pharmacotherapy for smoking cessation. Drugs. 2000;59:17-31

[69] Hughes JR, Goldstein MG, Hurt RD, Shiffman S. Recent advances in the pharmacotherapy of smoking. *JAMA.* 1999;281:72-6

[70] Paperwalla KN, Levin TT, Weiner J, Saravay SM. Smoking and depression. Med Clin North Am 2004;88:1483-94,x--xi

[71] Quattrocki E, Baird A, Yurgelun-Todd D. Biological aspects of the link between smoking and depression. *Harv. Rev. Psychiatry.* 2000;8:99-110.

[72] Siu ECK, Tyndale RF. Non-Nicotinic Therapies for Smoking Cessation. *Annu. Rev. Pharmacol. Toxicol.* 2007;47:541-4

[73] Cooper BR, Wang CM, Cox RF, Norton R, Shea V, Ferris RM. Evidence that the acute behavioural and electrophysiological effects of Bupropion are mediated by a noradrenergic mechanism. *Neuropsychopahrmacology.* 1994;11:133-41.

[74] Freyer JD, Lukas RJ. Non competitive functional inhibition at diverse, human nicotinic acetylcholine receptor subtypes by bupropion, phencyclidine, and ibogaine. *J. Pharmacol. Exp. Ther.* 1999;288:88-92

[75] Slemmer JE, Martin BR, Damaj MI. Bupropion is a nicotinic antagonist. *J. Pharmacol. Exp. Ther.* 2000;295:321-27

[76] Hsyu PH, Singh A, Giargiari TD, Dunn JA, Ascher JA, Johnston JA. Pharmacokinetics of bupropion and its metabolites in cigarette smokers versus nonsmokers. *J. Clin. Pharmacol.* 1997;37:737-43

[77] Ahluwalia JS, Harris KJ, Catley D, Okuyemi KS, Mayo MS. Sustained release Bupropion for smoking cessation in African Americans: a randomized controlled trial. *JAMA*. 2002;288:468-74

[78] Aubin HJ, Lebargy F, Berlin I, Bidaut-Mazel C, Chemali-Hudry J, Lagrue G. Efficacy of Bupropion and predictors of successful outcome in a sample of French smokers: a randomized placebo-controlled trial. *Addiction.* 2004;99:1206-18.

[79] Hurt RD, Sachs DP, Glover ED, Offord KP, Johnson JA et al. A comparison of sustained-release Bupropion and placebo for smoking cessation. *N. Engl. J. Med.* 1997;337:1195-1202

[80] Swan GE, McAfee T, Curry SJ, Jack LM, Javitz H et al. Effectiveness of Bupropion sustained release for smoking cessation in a health care setting:a randomized trial. *Arch. Intern. Med.* 2003;163:2337-44

[81] Tonnesen P, Tonstad S, Hjalmarson A, Lebargy F, Van Spiegel PI et al. A multicentre, randomized, double-blind, placebo-controlled, 1 year study of Bupropion SR for smoking cessation. *J. Intern. Med.* 2003;254:184-92

[82] Jorenby DE, Leischow SJ, Nides MA, Rennard SI, Johnston JA, Hughes AR et al. A controlled trial of sustained release bupropion, a nicotine patch, or both for smoking cessation. *N. Engl. J. Med.* 1999;340:685-91

[83] US Food and Drug Administration. http://www.fda.gov/Drugs/DrugSafety/PostmarketDrugSafetyInformationforPatientsandProviders/DrugSafetyInformationforHeathcareProfesionals/ucm169986.html (Last accessed on 2nd May, 2010)

[84] Roddy E. Bupropion and other non-nicotine pharmacotherapies. *BMJ.* 2004;328:509-11

[85] US Food and Drug administration. FDA Approves Novel Medication for smoking cessation. http://www.fda.gov/bbs/topics/NEWS/2006/NEW01370.html (Last accessed April 14,2010)

[86] Tutka P, Zatonski W. Cytisine for treatment of nicotine addiction: From a molecule to therapeutic efficacy. *Pharmacol. Rep.* 2006;58:777-798.

[87] Kaur K, Kaushal S, Chopra SC. Varenicline for smoking cessation: A Review of the literature. *Curr. Ther. Res. Clin. Exp.* 2009;70:35-54

[88] Jainski DR, Preston KL. Assessment of dezocine for morphine-like subjective effects and miosis. *Clin. Pharmacol. Ther.* 1985;38:544-48.

[89] Busto U, Kaplamn HL, Zawertailo L, Sellers EM. Pharmacologic effects and abuse liability of bretazenil, diazepam and alprazolam in humans. *Clin. Pharmacol. Ther.* 1994;55:451-463.

[90] Obach SR, Reed-Hagen AE, Suzanne SK, Obach BJ, O'Connell TN, Zandi KS. Metabolism and disposition of varenicline, a selective $\alpha_4\beta_2$ acetylcholine receptor partial agonist, in vivo and in vitro. *Drug Metabolism and Disposition.* 2006;34:121-130

[91] Faessel HM, Gibbs MA, Clark DJ, Rohrbacher K, Stolar M, Burstein AH. Multiple dose pharmacokinetics of the selective nicotinic receptor partial agonist, varenicline, in healthy smokers. *J. Clin. Pharmacol.* 2006;46:1439-48

[92] Jorenby DE, Hays T, Rigotti NA, Azoulay S, Watsky EJ, Williams KE et al. Efficacy of varenicline, an $\alpha_4\beta_2$ Nicotinic acetylcholine Receptor Partial agonist vs Placebo or Sustaiend- Release Bupropion for smoking cessation: A Randomized Controlled Trial. *JAMA.* 2006;296:56-63.

[93] Gonzales D, Rennard SI, Nides M, Oncken C, Azoulay S, Billing CB, Watsky EJ, Gong J, Williams KE and Reeves KR. Varenicline, $\alpha_4\beta_2$Nicotinic Acetylcholine Receptor Partial agonist, vs Sustained – Release Bupropion and Placebo for smoking cessation: A Randomized Controlled trial. *JAMA.* 2006;296:47-55

[94] Tonstad S, Tonnesen P, Hajek P, Williams KE, Billing CB, Reeves KR. Effect of maintenance therapy with varenicline on smoking cessation: a randomized controlled trial. *JAMA.* 2006;296:64-71

[95] Cahill K, Stead LF, Lancaster T. Nicotine receptor partial agonists for smoking cessation. Cochrane Database of Systemic Reviews 2008;3:CD006103

[96] US FDA. http://www.fda.gov/Drugs/DrugSafety/Postmarket DrugSafety InformationforPatientsandProviders/ucm106540.htm (Last accessed on 2nd May, 2010)

[97] Cahill K, Stead L, Lancaster T. A preliminary benefit-risk assessment of varenicline in smoking cessation. *Drug Saf.* 2009;32:119-35

[98] Gunnell D, Irvine D, Wise L, Davies C, Martin RM. Varenicline and suicidal behavior: a cohort study based on data from the general practice research database. *BMJ.* 2009;3339:b3805

[99] Glassman AH, Jackson WK, Walsh BT, Roose SP, Rosenfeld Bl. Cigarette craving, smoking withdrawal, and clonidine. *Science.* 1984;226:864-6

[100] Covey LS, Glassman AH. A meta-analysis of double-blind placebo-controlled trials of clonidine for smoking cessation. *Br. J. Addict.* 1991;86:991-8

[101] Gourlay SG, Benowitz NL. Is clonidine an effective smoking cessation therapy? *Drugs.* 1995;50:683-690

[102] Gourlay SG, Stead LF, Benowitz NL. Clonidine for smoking cessation. *Cochrane Database Syst. Rev.* 2004;2:CD000058

[103] Glassman AH, Stetner F, Walsh BT, Raizman PS, Fleiss JL, Cooper TB et al. Heavy smokers, smoking cessation, and clonidine: results of a double blind, randomized trial. *JAMA.* 1998;259:2863-6

[104] Hilleman DE, Mohiuddin SM, Delcore MG, Lucas BD. Randomized controlled trial of transdermal clonidine for smoking cessation. *Ann. Pharmacother.* 1993;27:1025-8

[105] Prochazka AV, Weaver MJ, Keller RT, Freyer GE, Licari PA, Lofaso D. A randomized trial of nortriptyline for smoking cessation. *Arch. Intern. Med.* 1998;158:2035-39.

[106] Hall SM, Reus VI, Munoz RF, Sees KL, Humfleet G, Hartz DT et al. Nortriptyline and cognitive-behavioral therapy in the treatment of cigarette smoking. *Arch. Gen. Psychiatry.* 1998;55:683-90

[107] Prochazka AV, Kick S, Steinburnn C, Miyoshi T, Fryer GE. A randomized trial of nortriptyline combined with transdermal nicotine for smoking cessation. *Arch. Intern. Med.* 2004;164:2229-33

[108] Hughes JR, Stead LF, Lancaster T. Nortriptyline for smoking cessation: a review. *Nicotine Tob. Res.* 2005;7:491-99

[109] Melero A, Garrigues TM, Alos M, Kostka KH, Lehr CM, Schaefer UF. Nortriptyline for smoking cessation: release and human skin diffusion from patches. *Int. J. Pharm.* 2009;378:101-7

[110] Escobaz- Chavez JJ, Merino V, Lopez-Cervantes M, Rodriguez- Cruz IM, Quintanar- Guerrerro D, Ganem-Quintanar A. The use of iontophoresis in the administration of nicotine and non-nicotine drugs through the skin for smoking cessation. *Curr. Drug Discov. Technol.* 2009;6:171-85

[111] Pentel P, Malin D. A Vaccine for Nicotine dependence: Targeting the Drug rather than the brain. *Respiration.* 2002;69:193-97

[112] de Villers SHL, Lindblom N, Kalayanov G, Gordon S, Malmerfelt A, Johansson AM, Svensson TH. Active Immunization against nicotine suppresses nicotine-indiced dopamine release in the rat nucleus accumbens shell. *Respiration.* 2002;69:247-53

[113] Hatsukami DK, Rennard S, Jorenby D, Fiore M, Koopmeiners J, de Vos A et al. Safety and immunogenicity of a nicotine conjugate vaccine in current smokers. *Clin. Pharmacol. Ther.* 2005;78:456-67

[114] Heading CE. Drug evaluation: CYT-002-NicQb, a therapeutic vaccine for the treatment of nicotine addiction. *Curr. Opin. Investig. Drugs.* 2007;8:71-7

[115] Celtic Pharma. Celtic Pharma completes rapid enrollment in phase IIb study for TA-NIC, the nicotine vaccine for smoking cessation. Available from URL: http://www.celticpharma.com/news/ pr/release_ 102907.pdf [accessed 2010, April 15]

[116] Maurer P, Bachmann MF. Vaccination against nicotine: an emerging therapy for tobacco dependence. *Expert Opin. Investig. Drugs.* 2007;16:1775-83.

[117] Pentel PR, Malin DH, Enniffar S, Hieda Y, Keyler DE, Lake JR et al. A nicotine conjugate vaccine reduces nicotine distribution to brain and attenuates its behavioral and cardiovascular effects in rats. *Pharmacol. Biochem. Behav.* 2000;65:191-98

[118] Keyler DE, LeSage MG, Dufek MB and Pentel PR. Chnages in maternal and fetal nicotine distribution after maternal administration of monoclonal nicotine specific antibody to rats. *Int. Immunopharmacol.* 2006;6:1665-72

[119] Roiko SA, Harris AC, Keyler DE, LeSage MG, Zhang Y, Pentel PR. Combined active and passive immunization enhances the efficacy of immunotherapy against nicotine in rats. *JPET.* 2008;325:985-93

[120] Tanda G, Pontieri FE, Di Chiara G. Cannabinoid and heroin activation of mesolimbic dopamine transmission by a common mu 1 opioid receptor mechanism. *Science.* 1997;276:2048-50

[121] French ED. Delta9-Tetrahydrocannabinol excites rat VTA dopamine neurons through activation of cannabinoid CB1 but not opioid receptors. *Neurosci. Lett.* 1997;226:159-62

[122] Gonzalez S, Cascio MG, Fernandez-Ruiz J, Fezza F, Di Marzo V, Ramos JA. Changes in endocannabinoid contents in the brain of rats chronically exposed to nicotine, ethanol or cocaine. *Brain Res.* 2002;954:73-81

[123] Sanofi Aventis Pharmaceutical. http://en.sanofiaventis.com/binaries/ 20040309_acc_PDF_Acomplia_media_tcm28-14689.pdf Last accessed on April 13, 2010.

[124] Steinberg MB, Foulds J. Rimonabant for treating tobacco dependence. *Vasc Health Risk Manag.* 2007;3:307-11

[125] Sanofi Aventis Pharmaceuticals. http://en.sanofi-aventis.com/ binaries/20081105_rimonabant_en_tcm28-22682.pdf Last accessed on April 13, 2010.

[126] Tennant FS Jr., Traver AL, Rawson RA. Clinical evaluation of mecamylamine for withdrawal from nicotine dependence. *NIDA Res. Monger.* 1984;49:239-97

[127] Rose JE, Sampson A, Levin AD, Heningfield JE. Mecamylamine increase nicotine preference and attenuates nicotine discrimination. *Pharmacol. Biochem. Behavr.* 1989;32:933-38

[128] Rose JE, Behm FM, Westman EC, Levin ED, Stein RM, Rippika GV. Mecamylamine combined with nicotine skin patch facilitates smoking cessation beyond nicotine patch treatment alone. *Clin. Pharmacol. Ther.* 1994;56:86-99

[129] Rose JE, Behm FM, Westman EC. Nicotine-mecamylamine treatment for smoking cessation: the role of precessation therapy. *Exp. Clin. Psychopharmacol.* 1998;6:331-43

[130] Eissenberg T, Griffiths RR, Stitzer ML. Mecamylamine doesnot precipitate withdrawal in cigarette smokers. *Psychopharmacology.* 1996;127:328-36

[131] Rose JE, Behm FM, Westman EC. Brand-switching and gender effects in mecamylamine/nicotine smoking cessation treatment. In: 5th Annual Meeting of the Society for Research on Nicotine and Tobacco; 1999 March, 1999; San Diiego, US: Society for Research on Nicotine and Tobacco; 1999

[132] Zevin S, Jacob P 3rd, Benowitz NL. Nicotine-mecamylamine interactions. *Clin. Pharmacol. Ther.* 2000;68:58-65

[133] Benowitz NL, Jacob P. Metabolism of nicotine to cotinine studied by a dual stable isotope method. *Clin. Pharmacol. Ther.* 1994;56:483-93

[134] Messina ES, Tyndale RF, Sellers EM. A major role for CYP2A6 in nicotine C-oxidation by human liver microsomes. *J. Pharmacol. Exp. Ther.* 1997;282:1608-14

[135] Nakajima M, Kwon JT, Tanaka N, Zenta T, Yamamoto Y et al. Relationship between interindividual differences in nicotine metabolism and CYP2A6 genetic polymorphism in humans. *Clin. Pharmacol. Ther.* 2001;69:72-78

[136] Oscarson M, McLellan RA, Gullsten H, Yue QY, Lang MA et al. Characterisation and PCR-based detection of a CYP2A6 gene deletion found at a high frequency ina aChinese population. *FEBS Lett.* 1999;448:105-10

[137] Malaiyandi V, Lerman C, Benowitz NL, Jepson C, Patterson F, Tyndale RF. Impact of CYP2A6 genotype on pretreatment smoking behavior and nicotine levels from and usage of nicotine replacement therapy. *Mol. Psychiatry.* 2006;11:400-9

[138] Rao Y, Hoffman E, Zia M, Bodin L, Zeman M, Sellers EM et al. Duplications and defects in the CYP2A6 gene: identification, genotyping, and in vivo effects on smoking. *Mol. Pharmacol.* 2000;58:747-55

[139] Schoedel KA, Hoffmann EB, Rao Y, Sellers EM, Tyndale RF. Ethnic variation in CYP2A6 and association of genetically slow nicotine metabolism and smoking in adult Caucasians. *Pharmacogenetics.* 2004;14:615-26

[140] Sellers EM, Dortok D, Tyndale RF. CYP2A6 inhibition increases plasma nicotine concentrations during nicotine patch and gum. *Clin. Pharmacol. Ther.* 2002;71:17

[141] Sellers EM, Kaplan HL, Tyndale RF. Inhibition of cytochrome P450 2A6 increases nicotine's oral bioavailability and decreases smoking. *Clin. Pharmacol. Ther.* 2000;68:35-43.

[142] David S, Lancaster T, Stead LF. Opiod antagonists for smoking cessation. Cochrane Database Syst Rev 2001;3:CD003086.

[143] David S, Lancaster T, Stead LF, Evins AE. Opioid antagonists for smoking cessation. *Cochrane Database Syst. Rev.* 2006;4:CD003086

[144] Somaxon pharmaceuticals. http://www.newsrx.com/newsletters/Law-and-Health-Weekly/2006-08-26/082120063331387LH.html (Last accessed on 21, April, 2010)

[145] Cinciripini PM, Tsoh PM, Wetter DW, Lam C, de Moor C, Cinciripini L et al. Combined effects of venlafaxine, nicotine replacement, and brief counseling on smoking cessation. *Exp. Clin. Psychopharmacol.* 2005;13:282-92

[146] Niaura R, Spring B, Boreelli B, Hedeker D, Goldstein MG, Keuthen N et al. Multicentre trial of fluoxetine as an adjunct to behavioral smoking cessation treatment. *J. Consult. Clin. Psychol.* 2002;70:887-96

[147] Saules KK, Schuh LM, Arfken CL, Reed K, Kilbey MM, Schuster CR.. Double blind placebo controlled trial of fluoxetine in smoking

cessation treatment including nicotine patch and cognitive-behavioral group therapy. *Am. J. Addict.* 2004;13:438-46

[148] Spring B, Wurtman J, Wurtman R, el-Khoury A, Goldberg H, McDermott J et al. Efficacies of dexfenfluramine and fluoxetine in preventing weight gain after smoking cessation. *Am. J. Clin. Nutr.* 1995;62:1181-7

[149] Pomerleau OF, Pomerleau CS, Morrell EM et al. Effects of fluoxetine on weight gain and food intake in smokers who reduce nicotine intake. *Psychoneuroendocrinology.* 1991;16:433-40

[150] Killen JD, Fortmann SP, Schatzberg AF, Hayward C, Sussman L, Rothman M et al. Nicotine patch and paroxetine for smoking cessation. *J. Consult. Clin. Psychol.* 2000;68:883-9

[151] Berlin I, Said S, Spreux-Varoquaux O, Launay JM, Olivares R, Millet V et al. A reversible Monoamine Oxidase A inhibitor (moclobemide) facilitates smoking cessation and abstinence in heavy, dependent smokers. *Clin. Pharmacol. Ther.* 1995;58:444-52

[152] Sugita S, Johnson SW, North RA. Synaptic inputs to $GABA_A$ and $GABA_B$ receptors originate from discrete afferent neurons. *Neurosci. Let.* 1992;134:207-11

[153] Yim CY, Mogenson GJ. Electrophysiological studies of neurons in the ventral tegmental area of Tsai. *Brain Res.* 1980;181:301-13

[154] Kalivas PW, Churchill L, Klitenick MA. GABA and enkephalin projection from the nucleus accumbens and ventral pallidum to the ventral tegmental area. *Neuroscience.* 1993;57:1047-60

[155] Fattore L, Cossu G, Martellotta MC, Fratta W. Baclofen antagonizes intravenous self-administration of nicotine in mice and rats. *Alcohol. Alcohol.* 2002;37:495-8

[156] Paterson NE, Froestl W, Markou A. The GABAB receptor agonists baclofen and CGP44532 decreased nicotine self-administration in the rat. *Psychopharmacology.* (Berl) 2004;172:179-86

[157] Sofuoglu M, Mouratidis M, Yoo S et al. Effects of tiagabine in combination with intravenous nicotine in overnight abstinent smokers. *Psychopahrmacology.* (Berl) 2005;181:504-10

[158] Slotkin TA. If nicotine is a developmental neurotoxicant in animal studies, dare we recommend nicotine replacement therapy in pregnant women and adolscents? *Neurotoxicol. Teratol.* 2008;30:1-19

[159] Maritz GS. Are nicotine replacement therapy, varenicline or bupropion options for pregnant mothers to quit smoking? Effects on the respiratory system of the offspring. *Ther. Adv. Respir. Dis.* 2009;3:193-210

[160] Eisenberg MJ, Filion KB, Yavin D, Belisle P, Mottilo S, Joseph L et al. Pharmacotherapies for smoking cessation: a metaanalysis of randomized controlled trials. *CMAJ.* 179:136-43

[161] Prochazka AV, Kick S, Steinburg C, Miyoshi T, Fryer GE. A randomized trial of nortriptyline combined with transdermal nicotine for smoking cessation. *Arch. Intern. Med.* 2004;164:2229-33.

[162] Smith SS, McCarthy DE, Japuntich SJ, Christansen B, Piper ME, Jorenby De et al. Comparative effectiveness of 5 smoking cessation pharmacotherapies in primary care clinics. *Arch. Intern. Med.* 2009;169:2148-55

[163] Piper ME, Smith SS, Schlam TR, Fiore MC, Jorenby DE, Fraser D et al. A randomized placebo-controlled clinical trial of 5 smoking cessation pharmacotherapies. *Arch. Gen. Psychiatry.* 2009;66:1253-62

[164] Ebbert JO, Croghan IT, Sood A, Schroeder DR, Hays JT, Hurt RD. Varenicline and bupropion sustained-release combination therapy for smoking cessation. *Nicotine Tob. Res.* 2009;3:234-9.

[165] Glover ED, Laflin MT, Schuh KJ, Schuh LM, Nides M, Christen AG et al. A randomized, controlled trial to assess the efficacy and safety of a transdermal delivery system of nicotine/mecamylamine in cigarette smokers. *Addiction.* 2007;102:795-802

[166] Hall SM, Humfleet GL, Resus VI, Munoz RF, Cullen J. Extended nortriptyline and psychological treatment for cigarette smoking. *Am. J. Psychiatry.* 2004;161:2100-07.

INDEX

A

absorption, 5, 7, 13, 15, 19, 20, 22, 53, 54
abuse, 20, 23, 27, 52, 58
acetylcholine, 1, 52, 57, 58
actuation, 15
adhesives, 12
adolescents, vii
adverse event, 28, 33
African Americans, 57
aggression, 26
agonist, 27, 29, 45, 58
alcohol withdrawal, 29
allele, 39
alveoli, 23
ambient air, 19
ambient air temperature, 19
anorexia, 26
anorexia nervosa, 26
antibody, 33, 34, 60
antidepressant, 43
anxiety, 26, 29
apoptosis, 47
arousal, 5

B

bacteriophage, 33

behaviors, 1, 39
beneficial effect, 37
beverages, 7, 14, 19
bicarbonate, 13
bioavailability, 53, 55, 62
blood-brain barrier, 33
boredom, 8
brain, 1, 2, 33, 52, 59, 60
brainstem, 35
buccal mucosa, 7, 19
bulimia, 26

C

cancer, viii
cannabinoids, 35
carbon, 23, 39
carbon monoxide, 23
cardiovascular disease, viii, 32
caregivers, 28
cation, 27
Caucasians, 62
challenges, 22
China, 51
cigarette smoke, 22, 27, 29, 57, 61, 64
cigarette smokers, 27, 29, 57, 61, 64
cigarette smoking, 11, 19, 22, 23, 37, 53, 56, 59, 64
circulation, 15
clinical trials, 23, 28, 31, 33, 34, 45

CNS, 1, 37
cocaine, 60
coffee, 7, 14
cognition, 52
color, iv
combination therapy, 26, 31, 34, 49, 64
complexity, 19
compliance, 12
compounds, 35
constipation, 37
consumption, 19
controlled trials, 26, 59, 64
copyright, iv
correlation, 55
cortex, 1
cost, 34
cotinine, 39, 55, 61
cough, 14
coughing, 9, 17, 20
counseling, 56, 62
craving, 7, 12, 14, 15, 23, 29, 53, 54, 56, 59
cues, 2, 37
cytochrome, 62

D

damages, iv
database, 59
deaths, vii, 51
defects, 39, 62
delusions, 26
depression, 25, 26, 28, 31, 35, 56
desensitization, 2, 5
detection, 62
developed countries, vii
developing nations, vii
diabetes, 14
diffusion, 59
discrimination, 61
disorder, viii, 9
disposition, 58
distress, 14
dopamine, 1, 25, 27, 33, 43, 60
dopaminergic, 1, 25, 45
dosage, 1, 13, 20, 55
dosing, 5, 8, 13
drug delivery, 5
drug dependence, 33, 35, 52
drug interaction, 9, 10
drugs, 3, 6, 26, 28, 34, 47, 49, 59
dyspepsia, 8, 9, 14

E

emotional distress, 14
endorphins, 1
enrollment, 60
epidemic, vii, 3
epilepsy, 26
epinephrine, 1
ethanol, 60
exercise, 11, 54
experts, 51
exposure, 2, 7, 21, 35, 47

F

FDA, 3, 7, 10, 22, 26, 27, 28, 29, 57, 58
fetus, 47
filtration, 27
flatulence, 14
flexibility, 8
fluctuations, 20
fluoxetine, 43, 62, 63
food intake, 63
forebrain, 35

G

gender effects, 37, 61
genotype, 62
glutamate, 1
glycerol, 35
glycolysis, 47
group therapy, 63
guidelines, vii, 3, 47

H

half-life, 15, 27
hallucinations, 26
hazards, 51
headache, 9, 12, 14
heart disease, 14
heartburn, 9
hepatic necrosis, 26
heroin, 60
hippocampus, 1, 25, 35
hostility, 26
human brain, 1
hypersensitivity, 26
hypertension, 14, 29, 30

I

immunization, 33, 34, 60
immunogenicity, 60
immunotherapy, 60
in vivo, 55, 58, 62
incidence, 8, 12, 14, 22
India, vii, 51
inhaler, 3, 5, 9, 19, 20, 22, 24, 54, 55
inhibition, 39, 45, 47, 57, 62
inhibitor, 43, 63
insomnia, 9, 12, 26
interneurons, 45
intervention, 47
isotope, 61

K

kinetics, 27, 52

L

labeling, 22
later life, 47
litigation, vii
liver, 61

locus, 25
lung disease, viii

M

major depression, 31
majority, 39
mammalian brain, 1
management, 25, 47
mania, 26
marketing, 26
media, 55, 61
median, 22
medication, 7, 10, 11, 14, 15, 19, 23, 28, 29, 31
meta-analysis, 12, 14, 21, 24, 29, 49, 54, 59
metabolism, 3, 22, 27, 39, 61, 62
metabolites, 26, 57
mice, 34, 52, 63
microsomes, 61
midbrain, 1
miosis, 58
moclobemide, 43, 63
molecules, 3, 22, 33
mood change, 28
morphine, 58
mortality rate, vii
mucosa, 7, 15

N

nausea, 9, 14, 28
negative consequences, viii
negative reinforcement, viii, 5
neurons, 1, 25, 45, 60, 63
neurotransmission, 45, 47
neurotransmitter, 47
nonsmokers, 12, 57
non-smokers, 26
norepinephrine, 43
nucleus, 45, 60, 63

O

oxidation, 61

P

parallel, 21, 43
paranoia, 26
parenchyma, 47
paroxetine, 63
PCR, 62
peptides, 41
permission, iv, 16
pharmaceuticals, 62
pharmacokinetics, 11, 26, 33, 39, 54, 55, 56, 58
pharmacological treatment, 25
pharmacotherapy, 3, 5, 47, 49, 51, 53, 56
phencyclidine, 57
phenytoin, 9
placebo, 6, 13, 15, 19, 21, 26, 27, 29, 33, 35, 39, 41, 43, 49, 54, 57, 59, 62, 64
placenta, 47
pleasure, 6
polymorphism, 61
polyps, 17
population growth, vii
positive reinforcement, 5
postural hypotension, 30
potassium, 13
prevention, 28, 34
priming, 34
probability, 21
proliferation, 47
properties, 45, 52
Pseudomonas aeruginosa, 33
psychiatric illness, 10, 28
psychobiology, 53
psychosis, 26

R

rash, 26

reactions, 12
reactive airway disease, 17
reactivity, 33
receptors, 1, 2, 5, 25, 33, 35, 47, 52, 60, 63
recombination, 33
recommendations, iv
reinforcement, viii, 2, 5, 52
relapses, 21
relief, 23, 53, 54, 55
renal failure, 27
replacement, 5, 53, 54, 55, 56, 62, 63
rhinitis, 9, 17, 20
rhinorrhea, 17
rights, iv
risk assessment, 58

S

saturation, 2
secretion, 27
seizure, 26
selective serotonin reuptake inhibitor, 25, 43
sensation, 8, 14, 17
sensitivity, 9
serotonin, 1, 31, 43
serum, 20, 26, 34
side effects, 14, 17, 26, 31
signals, 1
Singapore, 52
sinusitis, 17
skin, 12, 26, 59, 61
sleep disturbance, 10
smoking cessation, viii, 3, 5, 9, 19, 20, 21, 23, 25, 26, 27, 28, 29, 31, 34, 35, 37, 39, 41, 43, 45, 47, 49, 51, 54, 55, 56, 57, 58, 59, 60, 61, 62, 63, 64
sodium, 13
Spring, 62, 63
stimulus, 7, 23
strategy, 21, 33, 39
striatum, 35
success rate, 14, 21

suicidal behavior, 59
suicidal ideation, 26, 28
suicide, 26, 28
surface layer, 11
susceptibility, 47
symptoms, 2, 5, 8, 9, 11, 12, 14, 15, 25, 26, 27, 28, 29, 37, 55
syndrome, 29

T

target population, 49
temperature, 19
therapeutics, 52
therapy, 5, 7, 12, 14, 21, 23, 25, 29, 31, 43, 49, 53, 54, 55, 56, 58, 59, 60, 61, 62, 63
thoughts, 28
tin, 8, 14
tobacco, vii, viii, 1, 3, 5, 6, 7, 11, 15, 17, 29, 31, 34, 41, 43, 49, 51, 53, 60, 61
tobacco smoke, viii
tobacco smoking, vii, 5
toxicity, 23
transmission, 60
trial, 11, 13, 19, 21, 23, 35, 37, 43, 54, 55, 57, 58, 59, 62, 64
tricyclic antidepressant, 25, 31
tricyclic antidepressants, 25, 31
tuberculosis, 51

U

urinary retention, 31
urine, 25, 27

V

vaccine, 33, 60
vapor, 55
variations, 39
venlafaxine, 62
vision, 31

W

waking, 13, 14
wear, 11
weight gain, 8, 43, 63
withdrawal, viii, 2, 5, 8, 9, 11, 12, 14, 15, 25, 26, 27, 28, 29, 34, 37, 53, 54, 55, 59, 61
World Health Organisation, 51

Y

young adults, vii, 49